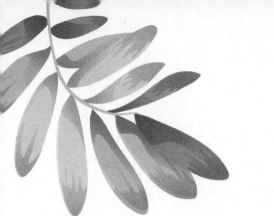

SUPER
AGER

Published by Mango Publishing Group, a division of Mango Media Inc.

Cover, Layout & Design: Morgane Leoni

For permission requests, please contact the publisher at:

Mango Publishing Group
2850 Douglas Road, 3rd Floor
Coral Gables, FL 33134 U.S.A.
info@mango.bz

For special orders, quantity sales, course adoptions and corporate sales, please email the publisher at sales@mango.bz. For trade and wholesale sales, please contact Ingram Publisher Services at:
customer.service@ingramcontent.com or +1.800.509.4887.

Super Ager: You Can Look Younger, Have More Energy, a Better Memory, and Live a Long and Healthy Life

Library of Congress Cataloging
ISBN: (p) 978-1-63353-738-5, (e) 978-1-63353-739-2
Library of Congress Control Number: 2018939403
BISAC - HEA049000 — HEALTH & FITNESS / Longevity

Printed in the United States of America

SUPER AGER

You Can Look **Younger**,
Have More **Energy**,
A Better **Memory**
and Live a **Long**
and Healthy **Life**

ELISE MARIE COLLINS

Mango Publishing
CORAL GABLES

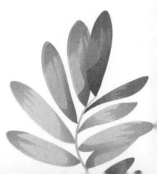

I want to thank my parents, Marie and Leonard, who taught me to never stop striving. I dedicate this book to the memory of my grandparents, who taught me to Super Age: Mama, Papa, Louise, and George. Thank you to my son Krishna for your support and understanding. I also thank my action partner Jean, Cate Stillman, and the Yogahealer community. May you be happy, may you be healthy, may you be at peace.

CONTENTS

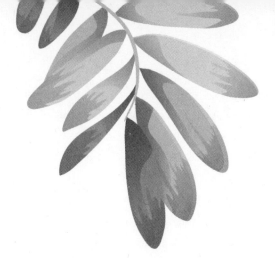

FOREWORD

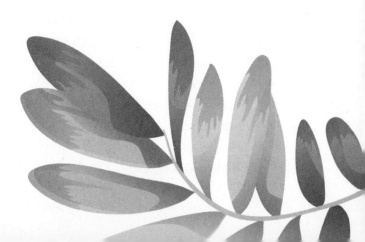

When Elise told me her book was titled *Super Ager*, I was ignorant that there was a term, even a concept, by that name. I was also ignorant of the research regarding the Blue Zones®. My initial reaction was to contract. My mind skipped the "super" and went straight to "ager." *How is she going to sell a book with the word "ager" in it*, I thought.

Super Ager, like Elise, is bold, brave, innovative, and sweet. Rather than shying away from our cultural aversion to aging, she goes into the heart of what is happening in these tiny pockets around the planet where our human elders are thriving into their eighties, nineties, and beyond. Elise shares the stories of these Super Agers, in their voices, in their cultures, so these experiences of common, everyday Super Agers ignite *your* vision for *your* future.

If you're a smart cookie, you'll read each and every page of this book. You'll keep it as a scientific reference guide and a go-to source of spiritual and inspirational wisdom to direct your personal aging process.

The fundamental question you will come back to as you read *Super Ager* is this: *how do you want to play your aging game?* Elise is a wise, modern-day yogi, practicing jnana yoga. She enlightens through innovative, inspirational wisdom that stimulates you into aligned action.

You too can be a Super Ager.

You are in the driver's seat, making small choices daily that compound into your aging future. *Super Ager* awakens you to discover how you want to do *your* aging. Elise scientifically explains the rules of the game if you want to be a Super Ager—if you want to thrive into your later decades—if you want to experience the connectivity possible for you as a human being, in your decades ahead.

Elise explains what is working for Super Agers and why, through the lens of Ayurveda, the holistic wisdom tradition that co-arose with yoga as the path to radiant longevity and everyday growth. I've devoted my career to sharing Ayurvedic wisdom, and Elise has been a partner on my path as the editor of our *Yoga Health Coaching* blog. Her generous heart and brilliant mind consistently escort me to new ways of thinking. In *Super Ager*, she has created a boon for Yoga Health Coaches and wellness pros from all traditions, to guide our society in thriving together.

As you read *Super Ager*, you will re-inspire yourself in the ancient truths about how we age, and discover what is possible for you. You will stimulate the path you must take to evolve right now and into who you truly want to be.

No joke.

You know there is room for you to grow smarter, more fun, more in the flow, and more connected.

If you want to be continually thriving with each day and each decade, get a few pals together—and start a *Super Ager* book club. Be smitten by your potential. Evolve together as a core Super Ager strategy.

CATE STILLMAN
Founder of Yogahealer and Yoga Health Coaching

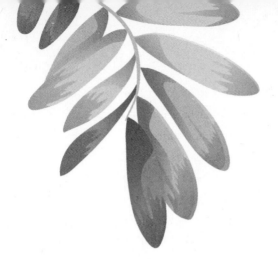

INTRODUCTION

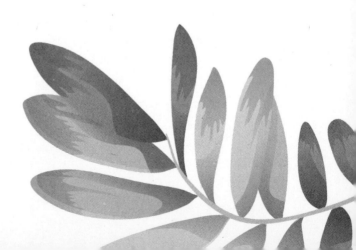

How you age is based mostly on what you do on a daily basis, and this biological fact remains true all throughout life. No matter how many candles are on your birthday cake, it is always possible to change how you are aging. By conservative estimates, 75 percent of how we age depends on lifestyle, not genetics—and even this genetic component is not set in stone! Changing how you live changes the way your genes express themselves in your body, through an "on/off switch" phenomenon called "epigenetics." Our genes can act differently, depending on the way we act and behave, the way think and believe, and even the way we view and handle our social and environmental circumstances. Epigenetics is still somewhat of a mystery, but some scientists believe that we will someday be able to influence over 90 percent of what our genes do! This optimism may be premature, but the emerging field of epigenetics promises to give us even greater control over our longevity and health. And since daily behavior already accounts for 75 percent or more of how you age, the opportunities are vast. You *can* Super Age.

While it's true that there is no exact formula on how to live to one hundred, your activities, the food you eat, how much you sleep, how you move, who you see, how you view your life, and more have massive impacts on how you age. To Super Age means to slow down your relationship with time, to grow younger, and to grow older more slowly. The good news is that Super Aging is more accessible than ever before. With the right tools and knowledge, you can Super Age with ease. And because each person is unique, the recipe for Super Aging is as individual as each human. *Super Ager* will teach you to tune in to your inner knowledge of what works for you. You will start with the simplest baby step, and then make small changes—changes that meet you where you are *currently* at—in order to Super Age. You will be inspired by Super Agers such as Tao Porchon-Lynch, a 99-year old-yoga teacher who once marched with Gandhi, or Whang-od Oggy, a 101-year-old traditional tattoo artist living in the Philippines, or

Virginia McLaurin, a 109-year-old who spins basketballs with the Harlem Globetrotters and has danced with the Obamas. You will uncover doable steps to extend your life and create an even better life for yourself right now. These steps are not chemicals or pills, although your chemistry does go along with your behavior. The steps that you take to optimize your life and to use "slow-down time" will also enhance your life. Super Aging may not always cause you to live longer, because life holds no guarantees, but the steps you take will always cause you to live more fully. You will learn to get together more often with friends, eat more plants, take more classes, play more, dance more, see more sunrises, and feel more satisfaction with your life. The best-kept secret is that there are so many ways to slow down the paths to aging, many of which are lots of fun. This book presents simple, easy-to-follow tips and tricks taken from Ayurveda, the world's oldest holistic healing modality. Each will give you tips and tricks to Super Age. Finally, this book enables you to build your Super Ager plan, a vision of organic growth through a plan of deliberate action and new habits. You will decide what you will do to Super Age. Use this book as your guide to change old habits and lifestyle choices into habits of Super Agers. Start by changing easier things first. As your confidence grows, you can say, "I got this." Soon you may find yourself taking on more challenging routines to increase your lifespan and your health span. You may even change behaviors that you never dreamed you would reverse. It's all up to you. In the end you will write your plan for life as a Super Ager, and you will think of your life as a beautiful garden that you will plant, prune, weed, and care for daily. Get ready: the time is now, so get set to Super Age!

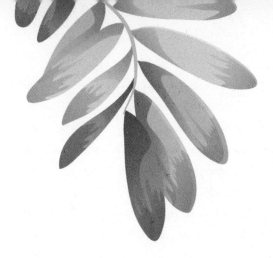

CHAPTER 1

What Is a Super Ager and How Can I Become One?

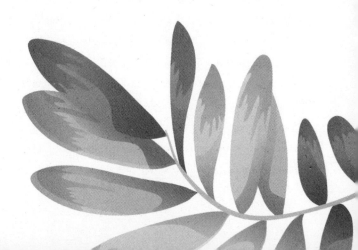

Do you want to look great, feel fabulous, and stay fit as you age? Why not have the best times of your life as you grow older? What if you could have an eternally youthful and positive attitude as the years roll by? What if your mindset could help you feel more vibrant than people half your age? Are you ready to shift towards this new possibility? That potential is called Super Aging and it is much closer than you think. You have heard the phrase, "Age is just a number." At this time in history, that motto has never been more true. You have a tremendous opportunity to disrupt and transform how you age. Are you doing it? Even the World Health Organization states: "Health in older age is not random." Are you living up to your aging potential? In these pages, you will find inspiration, tips, and tools to change the way you live and the way you age. Prepare to Super Age.

What is a Super Ager? The concept has been attributed to Dr. Marsel Mesulam, a cognitive neurologist who used the term to describe older adults who had the memory skills and attention spans typical of individuals several decades younger. Middle-aged Super Agers studied by Northeastern University showed that it is possible to have the brainpower of a twenty-seven-year-old, even when you're sixty-four. Other studies have demonstrated instances where adults aged eighty and older still have the cognitive ability of someone half their age. In recent years, the term "Super Ager" has been used to describe older adults who demonstrate the brainpower of someone many years younger, but the Super Ager concept is broader, and includes those older adults who have the athletic ability, creativity, inspiration, looks, and spunk of someone two to six decades younger. *Approaching 100: Secrets of The Superagers*, a 2017 BBC News series, is just one example of a growing interest in the topic of quality longevity. Super Agers are athletes, professors, great-grandparents, yogis, artists, and scientists. They are older adults who express phenomenal agility, strength, compassion, mental acuity, resilience, and endurance. The number of Super Agers is increasing, and many scientists are studying them. Many observe that Super Agers are resilient, enjoy challenges, and are eager to set goals. A friend told me the story of his great-grandmother, who had been a farmer in rural China. In her later years, she resided in Northern California, where she was frequently seen mowing the lawn at age 105. Neighbors judged the family harshly for making this centenarian do family chores. The truth was that her active participation in her family life through mowing in the garden kept this great-grandmother feeling alive and contributing to her family and community. Super Agers just keep on mowing.

At this time in history, aging is changing around the globe. As the average global lifespan keeps increasing, the world's average person keeps getting older and older—and the shift towards older populations is itself speeding up. This exponential growth in average human lifespan means that as time goes on, questions of aging will increasingly become more and more relevant to society and its members. There's strength in numbers, and as more people age and get older, now is the time to overthrow old paradigms. In 1990, the number of centenarians worldwide was 95,000. By 2015, that number had quadrupled to 451,000. By 2050, the number of centenarians on earth will grow by 800 percent to over 3.5 million centenarians. Centenarians are just an extreme example of a larger trend: by 2050, the number of people on the planet over the age of sixty-five will double. This massive shift will not only change the way we age; I predict this group of people will change the history of the world. And we need these Super Agers. Overwhelming technological and cultural changes are turning the world upside down. Those who have lived a long and happy life of eighty to a hundred years have learned many lessons critical to our survival. In many cultures, elders are revered for their wisdom and knowledge. As we age globally, older adults can teach humanity the lessons of forgiveness, self-compassion, gratitude, and love. I believe the world will benefit from the growing numbers of older adults in the world.

"Madame Full Charge"

Barbara Graves was "a dedicated and determined human rights and anti-war activist," who died at the age of 104, in Mill Valley, California. Her friends knew her as "Madame Full Charge." She read the paper daily and looked for causes that she would champion. Before she turned 100, she told a friend, "I don't want to be 100, because then I'll just be remembered for being 100." I want to acknowledge Barbara Graves for her accomplishments and her legacy. She led humanitarian programs in Tanzania, Haiti, Guatemala, and India. She was a tireless advocate for the environment and the underserved, an unforgettable human being who truly made a difference. By the year 2050, there will be eight times the number of centenarians alive on the planet as are today. When living to 100 becomes less unusual, we will remember Barbara Graves not only for her age, but for all she added to the world. And imagine if there were eight women like her daily fighting worldwide injustices for over 100 years.

Research into how to end aging is not new. Many ancient cultures had formulas, systems, and practices to extend life. Yet in the past few decades, scientific discoveries have revealed promising possibilities for life extension. Experimentation and discoveries have been converging at a rapid and exponential pace. The aging process in humans remains incredibly complex, yet multiple discoveries relating to various aging pathways have made the idea of ending aging seem possible. Companies such as Google's Calico, SENS research, and The Longevity Fund (a venture capital firm) all are racing to slow the paths of aging. Biologists have extended the life of a worm by ten times. A team of scientists have doubled the life expectancy of prematurely aging mice. But what does this mean for humans? We don't know yet. Could you live to be two hundred? Maybe. Could aging naturally become a fashionable trend a century from now? No one knows exactly what the future will bring, but you can bet that medical and health breakthroughs will keep on coming at the rapid pace of a high-speed video game.

The World's Oldest Yoga Teacher

The world's oldest yoga teacher, Tao Porchon-Lynch, ninety-nine, marched with Gandhi when she was ten years old. Raised by her aunt and uncle in Pondicherry, India, she's been called a real-life Forrest Gump because of her magical life. When Tao was eight, she saw young boys playing what she thought was a new game. It looked fun, so she joined them. It was actually yoga, and even though her aunt told it was just for boys, she insisted on learning it. As a lifelong passion, yoga was intertwined with her life. She worked as a model and film actress, and she met numerous celebrities and world leaders. In the 1950s, she taught yoga to Hollywood notables. The list of yoga teachers that Tao Porchon-Lynch has studied with sounds like a who's who of modern yoga: Sri Aurobindo, B. K. S. Iyengar, Pattabhi Jois, Swami Prabhavananda, Maharishi Mahesh Yogi. In 1967, she abandoned acting to become a full-time yoga teacher. Tao's words and positive spirit shine forth in her 2014 TED Talk, "You Can Do Anything." At age ninety-nine, she sits comfortably in lotus position, bending her legs like a pretzel, but more impressive is her indomitable spirit. At age eighty-seven, she took up ballroom dancing, especially tango, and has won over six hundred first-place awards. She inspires the world and reminds us to turn to nature for inspiration: "Use the wonderful laws of nature to recycle your whole body. Nature gives us clues to living in trees that are hundreds of years old. If you realize the trees look dead and now they bloom. The trees are going through their recycling period." Tao Porchon-Lynch has had many setbacks in life, including three hip replacements. In 2018, she will turn 100 years old, and her inspiration and resilience to bounce back from setbacks and embrace life is truly exhilarating.

THE SCIENCE OF LIFE

Ayurveda is the original holistic age-stopping medicine. As one of the oldest integral healing system on the planet, Ayurveda means "science of life." It codifies how to live well and how to age well. Ayurveda has unique philosophical underpinnings that interweave everything from the food you eat, to your natural environment, to the phases of life. Ayurveda is a truly meta-holistic model of the world. In Ayurveda, the sister science to yoga, everything is interrelated. Because Ayurveda embraces all of life and nature with compassion, it can help you simplify the tangled and misinformed habits of industrialized societies. It is no accident that many places in the world where people routinely live to the age of 100 are cultures that never modernized. While we can't go back in time, Ayurveda can remind modern humans of the value of slowing down and mindfully connecting with nature. Researchers in the emerging field of circadian medicine are confirming the wisdom of Ayurvedic sages, who have long known that by attuning to the daily cycles of a twenty-four-hour day you can actually slow aging.

In Ayurveda, everything in the world can be separated into five elements: earth, water, fire, air, and ether. These elements are a part of you; they are in the food you eat; they are in the computers you type on. These elements are present everywhere, and their qualities can be seen in everything around you. Ayurveda arose from the wisdom of great sages and seers who spent most of their time in meditation and contemplation. These sages or *rishis* had the intuitive ability to tune in to the universe and humanity, and then reverse-engineer its creation to find out how diseases could be cured and how people could stay in good health and balance. The laws of physics can demonstrate how a musical instrument makes sound waves that humans experience as beautiful music. The laws of physics govern music and explain how it works. Ayurveda deciphers the music of the universe, and western science can explain how the sound waves of the universe operate. Together Ayurveda and science can help you to discover how you can optimize your own aging.

In Ayurveda, each stage of life has an element. All of the elements have qualities that explain the three stages of life. From birth to about sixteen years of age, you are in the earth and water stage of life. From sixteen years of age to about fifteen years, you are in the fire and air stage of life. From fifty to death, you are in the air and ether stage of life. When you know the elements of aging, you can find balance for yourself and use that balance to Super Age.

In the Ayurvedic model, each one of us is a completely unique blueprint. You are like a snowflake that has your own way of living, being, aging, and interacting with the world. While there is a genetic component to aging, our lifestyle accounts for 75 percent of our life expectancy. Ayurveda can teach you how to know yourself and optimize your own personal blueprint and physiology. When you are in balance, your physiology is optimized. To Super Age is to know yourself and to listen to your own inner wisdom. Scientists know how to help people live longer, yet only a small number of people are applying this information to their own lives. If we honor the idea that each age-slowing formula will be different from person to person, I believe people will change more easily. To Super Age is to meet yourself where you are and move in the right direction for you. There are people who drink whisky and live to be 111 years old. Some centenarians eat only whole foods, while others sometimes eat ice cream. And as Ayurveda teaches, we are each completely different. The key to Super Aging is careful personal investigation to find formulas and methods that work for you. What feels good to you? What will help you age and better yet, what will help you live life to the fullest and fulfill your dreams at 58, 67, 75, 84, 99 or 112? In *Super Ager* you will create a mosaic of daily habits and seasonal habits to optimize your own aging process.

TAKE CONTROL OF HOW YOU AGE

But isn't a lot of aging genetic? No, modest estimates measure genetics account for only 25 percent or less. The rest of the aging process—75 percent—is lifestyle. And lifestyle may even account for more; as the complex field of epigenetics grows, there is growing evidence that we influence our genome even more than previous thought.

If you are ready to take control of your life as a Super Ager, this book is for you. If you're fifty and over, this book will have many, many inspirational ideas and habits. If you are younger, you can put Super Ager habits in place and then coast through to middle age and beyond. There's a lot of wisdom here: whether you are sixty, seventy, eighty, or ninety-five, there's something for you here on these pages.

We need to learn preventative medicine based on good habits. As you will learn, contrary to popular belief, healthy habits are life-affirming, not rigid or boring. This is important because the medical system in the United States does not emphasize prevention. Americans spend more than any other country in the world per person per year on health care—about $10,348—yet we are ranked fifty-third in the world in life expectancy, at 79.25 years. In Japan, the average life expectancy is 85.52 years—more than six years longer than in the US—yet Japanese annual healthcare expenses, per person, are less than half of comparable American medical spending. More medical dollars does not mean more years of life. In Ikaria, Greece, modern "health care" is almost totally lacking. This isolated island has two doctors and a broken X-ray machine, yet it boasts the lowest middle-aged mortality rate in the world. In the last twenty years, demographers have defined "Blue Zones®" as areas in the world with significantly larger populations of centenarians. Almost all of the Blue Zones® don't have the economic prosperity of industrialized countries. Instead, members of many of the Blue Zone® communities remain self-reliant well into old age, despite poverty and lack of material success, and live an average of twelve extra years.

Enter the Blue Zone®

What is a Blue Zone®? A Blue Zone® is an area where statistically unusual numbers of verified centenarians live. There are five current Blue Zones®: Okinawa, Japan; The Nicoya Peninsula, Guatemala; Sardinia, Italy; Loma Linda, California; and Ikaria, Greece. Several of these regions are relatively isolated and remote, yet not all are places untouched by modern life. In these regions, people share the following common behaviors:

- Eat a plant-based diet.
- Engage in natural movements, such as walking, gardening, or other consistent physical exercise or movement.
- Have a sense of purpose.
- Belong to a community or faith-based community.
- Take family seriously.
- Practice the ability to relax, let go of worries, or downshift.
- Don't overeat or eat after sunset.

If you are in good health, you have opportunities right now to optimize the way you live and the way you age. Super Agers are people who step up from our hearts to shine and embrace our aging. What I have learned as a yoga teacher and Yoga Health Coach is that each one of us has a specific and unique way of living and aging. This book is about optimizing that process. When you optimize the way you're living, you optimize your life. Super Aging requires that you look at and let go of your limiting beliefs, so that you can to shift your habits and lifestyle for the better.

If you are ill or suffering from a chronic health condition, please check with your doctor before following any of the programs outlined in this book. Most of the suggestions in these pages are gentle and have little or no risk. Most suggestions are simple habits, activities, or recipes that are inexpensive and relatively easy to implement.

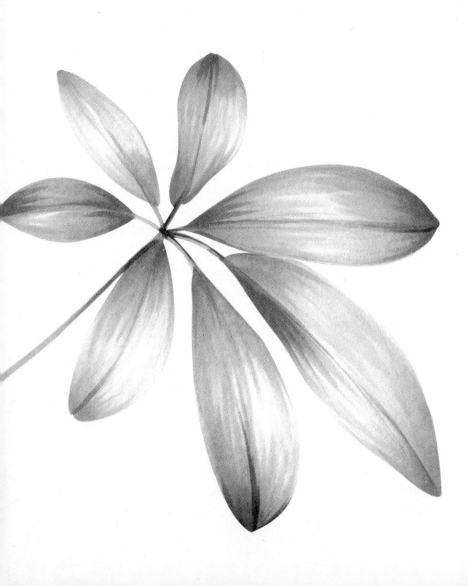

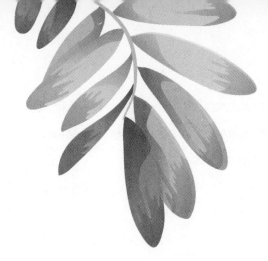

CHAPTER 2

Discover Your Foundation for Healthy Aging

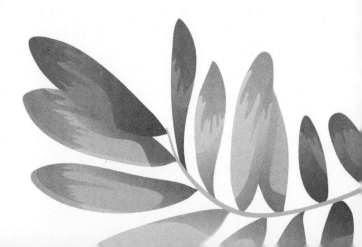

> **"You have to study yourself and what you want to do.**
> **You have a purpose, and that purpose has to be one**
> **that can change."**
>
> —Annie Mays Larmore (1907–2013), participant in the
> Georgia Centenarian Study

According to Ayurveda, the *Vata* (airy) stage of life begins at around age fifty. During this time of life, a new kind of wisdom evolves. We move from the Pitta (fiery) stage of life to the air portion of our journey. Western culture typically values the ego and power of the fire element over other qualities, making this transition tricky. Embracing the wisdom of our Vata years means letting go of our old identity and finding a new one. Chip Conley was fifty-two years old when Brian Chesky, one of the co-founders of Airbnb, asked Chip to become his mentor and help lead the growing startup. Back in the day, Chip had been an early "disruptor" of the hospitality industry. In the late '80s, he transformed a seedy, rent-by-the-hour motel with a pool in San Francisco into a go-to accommodation for touring rock bands, such as the *Red Hot Chili Peppers*. He grew a unique boutique hotel business called "Joie de Vivre," which had 3,500 employees when he sold it in 2010. A few years later, he was approached by Brian Chesky of Airbnb, who was wondering whether Chip would join the Airbnb team and mentor him. Chip was twice the age of the average employee at Airbnb and he would be reporting to a twenty-one-year-old. Even though he was all-in, he quickly realized that things were a bit different than he expected. By the end of his first week on the job, Chip explained to a friend, "I feel more like an intern than a mentor." In a team meeting, an engineer asked a question that, to someone unfamiliar with the tech, sounded like a Zen koan, "If we drop-ship an item to a customer and they don't use it, did it really drop-ship?" To get over the generation gap, Chip decided to emulate someone he admired greatly: anthropologist Margaret Mead. Pretending to be a cultural anthropologist was Chip's way of completely upending his own self-image in order to survive this new stage of his career and life. In his capacity at Joie de Vivre, he was superstar and CEO. While working at Airbnb, he would need to get over any and all of his addiction to admiration. He now advised behind the scenes. No longer would he be the guy with all the answers. Chip became curious: a hallmark quality of the Vata stage of life. His big transition meant letting go of the fire element of the ego and embracing the air element of older adulthood. The Vata time of life is all about wisdom, seeing the big picture, and connectedness. Intuitively, Chip aligned with the Ayurveda model of aging. He transitioned gracefully because he realized Airbnb did not need a second CEO going around spouting Baby-Boomer / Brick-and-Mortar wisdom to a bunch of people who wanted to reinvent hospitality. "I realized quickly I need to listen, with empathy and no ego and very little judgment." Going from center stage to coaching from the sidelines was not easy. It was the perfect movement from fire to air, from ego to wisdom. Chip Conley spent four years with Airbnb, helping them to grow exponentially. He has stayed on as an advisor to Airbnb because the company told him, "We can't exactly explain what you do for us, but your intangible value is critical to the company." This intangible value is exactly what describes the air element or Vata stage of life. It's all around, intangible, yet essential to life.

BECOME A MODERN ELDER

In the words of Chip Conley, a self-proclaimed "Modern Elder," there are a growing number of older adults who feel irrelevant. How do we create an intergenerational bridge? He likens the "Modern Elder,' someone who is someone who both serves and learns, is mentor and an intern and student and sage all at the same time. He thinks it is necessary for Boomers because we are going to live at least another ten years longer than our parents. We can create a way to learn from each other and connect generations. This wise advice comes from someone who has embraced the Vata stage of life.

Ayurveda Stages of Life

While science has no definitive model to explain aging or even why we age. There are a few animals, bacteria and plants that don't actually don't age. For thousands of years Ayurveda described life in three stages. From birth to puberty, the earth or Kapha stage of life: During this stage, children do a lot of growing. They are alive and full of earth. It is a time of attachment and love, nourishment. This is also why older generations and young children complement each other in balance. Babies are pure love and develop rapidly. Earth represents love and steadiness. Children teach us about nature and love as part of the earth element. Puberty to about age fifty is the Pitta or fire stage of life. In this stage of life, there is fire, ego, separation, sharpness. It is also a time of moving forward and accomplishment. The Pitta stage can transform. Teenage rebellion is a good example of the fire element. Watch out he/she is on fire, I would say of my own teenagers when they were in a particularly angry or righteous state. Professional sports and competition is the realm of fire. Fire, when out of balance destroys. Out of balance fire can also manifest as criticism directed at the self or others. Vata or air/ether stage of life is age fifty and up. These are the wisdom years of air. When we are high in the air, we can see the big picture. Air is inspiring and dominates the heart center. As the number of humans who are living in the Vata stage of life increases on the planet, I believe they will bring a much-needed breath of fresh "air." For the next few decades as the number of people over sixty-five doubles and the number of centenarians increases eight fold, the world will transform with more people in this inspirational heartfelt time of life. People who are in balance in the air stage of life offer considerable wisdom. People who are out of balance in the air stage of life become out of touch and disconnected

KEEP YOUR FIRE BURNING

Critical to Super Aging is finding one's purpose or reinventing one's purpose. A purpose not driven by ego, but by a deep desire. When you are younger, you have more of the fire element. Our drives and ambitions can have more of a fiery quality and when fire is out of balance, a person can be egoic and obnoxious. When you reach middle age, you must adjust, but not abandon your ambition and deep desires. Often purpose transforms to a desire to serve. Purpose becomes humbler and may be better described as contribution.

Chip Conley found his purpose in listening to and helping digital natives embrace emotional intelligence and leadership as they disrupted the hospitality industry. All generations gained wisdom and transferred information. When you find your purpose, you thrive in your able to meet adversity and face the challenges in your life, and especially those of aging. A purpose as we age is our passion and fire, it burns brightly and with strength. It helps to point us in the right direction to create a legacy, have better relationships or pursue a new vocation as an artist. Later in this chapter I will offer several styles of therapy or exploratory work that will be perfect for finding your passion and purpose.

Finding your purpose or reinventing your purpose is the at the heart aging in a healthy way. When you know your why, you can build a healthy life to support your why. Other words that may describe your purpose or your why could be contribution or service. If purpose sounds to lofty or goal oriented. Maybe asking the question, how can I serve the world right now in my life? Your answer may be different than it was ten or twenty or even thirty years ago. Don't be afraid to keep it simple. A grandfather named Tsegai told me that he drove Lyft for four to five hours a day to save money to give to his grandsons, ages seven and ten. He had retired from driving big rigs and running his own trucking business. He loved driving and he knew that his health depended on keeping busy. He set a goal to save a set amount for his grandsons. When he hits his mark, he told me he would like to serve young children in his community. He plans to volunteer to read and tutor elementary school children. He realized the importance of having goals and visions for his "retirement" years.

Your contribution or purpose may be to enjoy stimulating and wise conversations with friends and family. You may not be giving a TED Talk, but I know that if you have a purpose to have wise conversations, there will be a ripple effect. You will be gaining the health benefits of living your purpose and your purpose will in turn benefit the world. Your stimulating and inspiring conversations, if this is your purpose can embolden others young and old to come into their own powerful purpose.

Numerous studies have demonstrated that having a strong life purpose may help you dodge many debilitating conditions associated with aging. A 2017 study found that having a clear purpose had strong physiological effects on your health. In one study, people who reported having a purpose slept better and had less diagnosable sleep issues. Another study found a connection between those who reported feeling purposeful to having a faster gait and stronger grip strength. A study of older adults at Northwestern University defined purpose as, "having aspirations and goals for the future and feeling that experience in life are meaningful." People who reported having purpose have less sleep issues according to the study published in the July 2017 *Sleep Science and Practice Journal*. And subjects in this study were over 50 percent African American, a group that is often left out of research data yet suffer on average more sleep disturbances and a shorter life expectancy than white counterparts in the United States. The study found a link between purpose and better sleep over a long period of time. "Helping people cultivate a purpose in life could be an effective drug-free strategy to improve sleep quality, particularly for a population that is facing more insomnia" said the study's senior author, Jason Ong, professor of Neurology at Northwestern University Feinberg School of Medicine. "Purpose in life is something that can be cultivated and enhanced through mindfulness therapies," he added.

Finding a sense of purpose can add years to your life, according to a study at Canada's Carleton University. The researchers sorted through a long-term study of six thousand individuals over a fourteen-year period, looking to see if having a direction in life at any age affected longevity. The study concluded that greater purpose in life conferred benefits across lifespan and this was consistent even when other beneficial psychological traits were teased out ("correlation was not causation"). "These findings suggest that there's something unique about finding a purpose that seems to be leading to greater longevity," said lead researcher Patrick Hill. When you feel a desire to contribute to the world and have a personal connection to the value of that contribution to the world, you have a powerful health protector, one that is perhaps more potent than many pills.

IKIGAI: YOUR REASON FOR LIVING

The Japanese word *ikigai* can be translated in many ways. One simplified meaning can be "reason for living." For some this word may have more resonance than "purpose." The book, *Ikigai, The Japanese Secret to a Long and Happy Life*, by Hector Garcia and Francesc Miralles details the secret of ikigai and how the villagers of Ogimi, Okinawa (yes, that's within The Blue Zone® known as the "village of longevity") live their purpose, along with other helpful tips for readers who want to live a long and happy life. The book points out that there is no word for retirement in the Okinawan dialect, indicating that its culture values hard, yet joyous work in each stage of life. Many of the villagers in Ogimi describe their ikigai in practical words, "I plant my own vegetables and cook them myself. That's my ikigai." "Getting together with my friends is my most important ikigai. We all get together here and talk—it's very important. I always know I'll see them all here tomorrow, and that's one of my favorite things in life." Ikigai can also translate as "the happiness of always being busy" (Garcia and Miralles 2017). Indeed, ikigai infers deep connection and resonance to one's essential self. It seems related, yet not quite the same as the Sanskrit word dharma, a word that also has multiple meanings. Dharma can mean duty, a right way of living and when applied to an individual can confer "a purpose in life, independent of material pursuits." Getting to know oneself and what makes one joyful, as well as fulfilled would be of supreme importance in fulfilling dharma and ikigai as we grow older. In our search for meaning, we may discover new passions. Chip Conley, The Modern Elder recommends that a person become an expert in a subject that is interesting to them. He has become one of the world's experts in festivals, a subject that he finds fun and fascinating. Conley began pursuing this area of expertise by taking to heart the example of the late management guru Peter Drucker, who annually would learn and become an expert in one new subject: Drucker kept up his yearly expansion for over sixty years, long before modern neuroscience would affirm the wisdom of his perennial habit. The brain can indeed rewire and remold itself for the better even as we age, and even though neuroscience hadn't proved this yet, Drucker just kept on learning, all the way to age ninety-five.

One of the reasons that a deeper connection to inner purpose and *ikigai* later in life is important at any stage of life, but especially for older adults. When you are in touch with your own inner desire to contribute to the world, this quality balances the softer, vaguer nature of air that characterize the *Vata* stage of life. Your focus shifts as you age, and a healthy purpose is one that brings you joy. You may retire at age fifty-two to pursue painting and sculpting, or you may continue to work as a high school teacher or researcher when you are ninety-five; the critical element to healthy aging is feeling *connected* to something important to *you* and *your purpose*. Curiosity and intuition are hallmark qualities of air. We may long to be an "expert" or to do a lot of good. A study that analyzed data from ten previous studies involving 136,000 individuals in the United States and Japan found that people who reported a sense of purpose had a 20 percent lower risk of death and a lower rate of cardiovascular disease. It's important to note that if we have been fiery our entire life, we may need to soften during our Vata years to embrace a purpose that has a gentle quality. Desires are a gateway to our intuition and our true nature. Our desires become very important in midlife.

Our intuition and curiosity are very powerful internal compasses to help us connect with our *ikigai*. Follow those things you enjoy, and get away or change those you dislike. Be led by your curiosity and keep busy by doing the things that fill you with meaning and happiness. It doesn't need to be a big thing: we might find meaning in being good parents or in helping our neighbors.

Nicoya Peninsula of Guatemala: "Plan de Vida"

Indeed, each one of us, as Ayurveda reminds us, has a unique blueprint of elements and qualities which makes up our personality and our physiology in the world. When you connect to this deep blueprint, your life purpose will emerge naturally. Research demonstrates that a sense of purpose has positive aging benefits. One study showed that having a greater purpose predicted lower mortality. And a sense of purpose was measured independent of retirement status, which is a known risk for mortality. A life purpose outside of a "job" seems to have deep health-related benefits. It makes sense that once we know and understand our true purpose, we will feel like we want to take better care of ourselves and to be healthy.

In the Nicoya Peninsula of Guatemala, people have a "*plan de vida*," or reason to live. This "plan de vida" helps keep older adults active and positive in the face of adversity. Ayurveda can help us to bring more ease and less willfulness to our aging mindset. Air and ether gives perspective and wisdom. Air and ether also move erratically, we need more earth and fire to balance this Airy stage of life. When our lifestyle and our routine support us as we age, we can more easily choose a positive mindset. Think about when you feel calm and well-nurtured; when you feel frazzled and overwhelmed, it is hard to stay positive. This is when we need to step back and take a different approach. Ayurveda can give tremendous insight into aging, and especially how we age as individuals.

REFERENCES

Here are some references[1] that can help you flush out your *ikigai* or reason for living, especially if you feel blocked.

Therapy

- Research Logotherapy based on the work of Victor Frankl; www.logotherapyinstitue.org has more information and offers online classes.
- Morita Therapy has an extensive website based on Zen principles and extensive video resources at: www.moritaschool.com.

Books

- *Ikigai, The Japanese Secret to a Long and Happy Life* by Hector Garcia and Francesc Miralles
- *My One Chief Aim* by Mitch Horowitz
- *Wherever You Go, There You Are* by Jon Kabat-Zinn
- *The Desire Map,* by Danielle LaPorte
- *The Artist's Way,* by Julia Cameron
- *The Life-Changing Magic of Tidying Up,* by Marie Kondo
- *Your Inner GPS: Follow Your Inner Guidance to Health, Happiness and Satisfaction,* by Zen Cryar DeBrucke
- Also check out the Divine Purpose Meditation in Chapter 11

–PRACTICE PLAN–

- Journal Daily on your purpose or *ikigai*. Ask yourself question such as what brings me joy? Think about what you loved to do as a child or a teenager. What would you do if you could wave a magic wand and

---

1. There is also a bibliography at the end of the book.

be absolutely anything in the world? It is never too late to be an actor, dancer, writer, DJ, or an artist. Keep letting yourself dream.

- Be a detective for joy and purpose. Imagine that your reason for living is like a treasure. It could be far away, or it could be in plain sight. Get your mental magnifying glass and your spy kit and get to work. Remember your *ikigai* is unique and always, *always* inside of you.

- Read one of the recommended books and or start a Super Ager book group. Read books on purpose and discuss.

- Meditate – Meditators have a stronger sense of purpose, according to a study that followed meditators on retreat in Colorado. Following the retreat, meditators reported feeling a sense of meaning and purpose in life. If you have never meditated before, start with a small, daily practice. Use an app or a timer. Choose a time of day when you can meditate daily.

- If you do not feel strongly connected to your own reason for living, take a few hours a week to really seek your purpose. Spend these hours walking in nature, doing something fun that you might not usually allow yourself to do. Or go on an artist date. If you don't know what an artist date is, look up Julia Cameron and *The Artist's Way.*

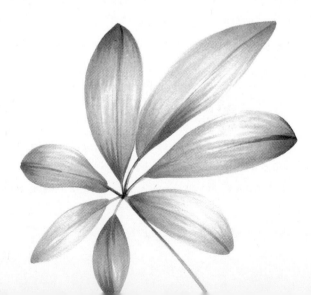

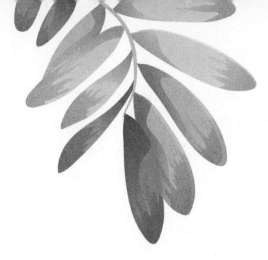

CHAPTER 3

See the World through Mindful Rose-Colored Glasses

"I never thought anything about age. I believe sincerely that there is nothing I can't do. All the power of the Universe is right inside of me."

—Tao Porchon-Lynch, yoga teacher, age ninety-nine

To Super Age is to embrace the power of the universe inside of you and to believe that your power is infinitely good. You will experience hardships, trials and tribulations throughout life. Successful aging means embracing these ups and downs and then choosing to see the good. This requires self-compassion and self-love. To pay attention to life, to see the beauty in each moment, is to see through mindful rose-colored glasses. Your health—mental, physical, spiritual and emotional—requires the digestion and assimilation of all life experiences. This requires great compassion towards yourself and others. In the purest sense, mindfulness actually means compassion. Mindfulness means paying attention with love. This is the greatest gift you can give yourself, your loved ones, and the world. When I listen to the stories and wisdom of the oldest of old, from nanogenerians to centenarians to super-centenarians, I hear compassion, gratitude, and acceptance. Sometimes a centenarian may seem feisty or crabby, but peel back the veneer, and deep compassion is present.

To embrace and live a long life, compassion towards yourself may be one of the most important tools. Compassion allows you to digest and integrate suffering. You will not be able to escape suffering, but you will be able to weave that pain into a beautiful tapestry called life. Once you have given yourself space for compassion, there is space for grief, for suffering, and for joy.

In every moment, you have a choice to see things as generally positive or negative. You may feel "negative" emotions such as anger, jealousy, fear, anxiety, judgment. Your health arises not from your ability to push away or shove these negative feelings into a corner or out of sight. Rather, it arises from giving these feelings space and a voice. Your resilience comes from quiet introspection and understanding all of the emotions and experiences of living. There is darkness and there is light. Healthy aging and longevity require deep wells of inner compassion. When you feel and not just pay lip service to that compassion, you are ready to move on to the next journey of life.

Yet life rarely presents clear forks in the road. Life is full of complexities and shades of gray. The brain or the mind has a job, and that is to keep us safe. Fear and negativity had a role in our evolution and survival. Vigilance and seeing things through a negative lens helped us survive at one point. Those who were fearful and vigilant survived more often than those who may have been more carefree. When humans anticipated a threat or attack and that was a correct assessment, negative thinking helped people to survive. As humans, we are always growing, learning, and watching out for danger. Our brains are wired to look for things to fear. But this is not the only way of looking at things. A positive outlook, even in the face of not so positive life circumstances, seems to be a personality trait that may be associated with longevity. And to survive eighty years and beyond, a certain kind of resilience and reframing will be necessary.

In 2017, Sardinians age 90–101 were interviewed about their life histories and beliefs. Younger relatives of this group of nano and octogenarians were also queried on their long-lived family members' personalities. Researchers found that these older adults exhibited better mental health than younger people. Despite a decline in physical vigor, older adults of Sardinia had a mostly positive outlook. They were filled with hope and optimism, despite what life had dealt them. It seems that to live to be 100, one either becomes more positive or perhaps optimism helps one survive past a certain age. In Ayurveda, the last part of life, is influenced by the air element which is expressed through a positive attitude and inspirational point of view.

Back to School

As one of the oldest undergraduates at UC–Berkeley, Delores Orr, age seventy, is part of a trend of older adults going back to college after age twenty-five. However, at her age, she is more of an exception at highly selective schools such as Berkeley. As Delores' own granddaughter struggled in elementary school, she told her grandma she believed she could not succeed in school. Delores Orr's pursuit of higher education arose from a deep desire to inspire her granddaughter. When her granddaughter continued to doubt that she could succeed in school, Delores told her, "but you can: I'll show you." She was accepted to Cal, yet when she arrived on the Berkeley campus, her confidence wavered. She found herself surrounded by students who looked and acted very different than her. They rode skateboards and stared at their smartphones. Orr felt her fear and then did something about it. She sat across from the office of the registrar at Sproul Hall, repeating positive affirmations over and over: "I am worthy, I am worthy, I am worthy." Her mindset leads her to her success. She will graduate in Spring of 2018.

THE POWER OF POSITIVE THINKING

Do optimists live longer than pessimists? Recent research suggests optimism strongly affects cardiovascular health. A 2015 University of Illinois study analyzed data from an ongoing survey, called the Multi Ethnic Study of Atherosclerosis, finding that those who exhibited the highest levels of optimism had almost double the odds of having ideal cardiovascular health, in comparison to their more pessimistic counterparts. The study's author, Rosalba Hernandez, Professor of Social Work at University of Illinois, emphasized that the significance of a hopeful attitude was clear. "This association remains significant, even after adjusting for socio-demographic characteristics and poor mental health," she said. In a similar study at Harvard University, researchers found links between optimism, hope, life satisfaction, and a reduced risk of cardiovascular disease, as well as strokes.

But can it be that easy? Believe it or not it can be, kind of. Affirmations can help redirect our neurons to create pathways that help override old and long-ingrained patterns. Breaking habitual patterns of negativity can be surprisingly easy and, well, hard. Why is that? Because the mind creates patterns, and breaking these patterns feels very, very uncomfortable. You are changing the neural pathways that direct the mind to fear. It is important to realize that this is very different than suppressing, overriding, or bypassing pain or reality. In the highest sense, when you feel the fear, name the fear, listen to the fear, express the fear, and give it compassion, you create space. Once you create this space, there is a potential to choose a new thought, a new goal, a new path, and this is the "positive" mindset that healthy aging both requires and (I believe) teaches. When we age in a healthy way, we become more resilient and we also become great teachers. There is potential in aging to learn deep lessons of resilience, and this imparts great wisdom on the person who is aging. This is the gift of Super Agers.

In Ayurveda, speaking, thinking, and acting in a way that is positive, kind, and truthful restores the spirit and the mind and helps increase feelings of wellbeing. A 2012 study revealed similar traits in centenarians. The study, titled "Positive attitude towards life and emotional expression as personality phenotypes for centenarians," included participants with an average age was 97.5 and found that "qualities of positivity," including being optimistic or easygoing, were more prevalent in the 243 centenarians studied than the average population in the US. Laughter was valued by these Super Agers, and most were part of a larger social network. Most were emotionally expressive, less neurotic, and expressed a higher-than-average level of conscientiousness. Similar studies of centenarians have evoked surprisingly likeminded data, indicating that perhaps the mental attitude of Super Agers contributes greatly to their ability to live so much longer than average.

The results of the Heidelberg Centenarian study challenged the belief that older adults have maxed out on feeling positive, given the adversities common in advanced age, such as losing a life partner or continual physical decline. Regardless of "accumulating negative conditions," the centenarians reported high levels of happiness and optimistic feelings on par with those of adults half of their age.

The Outside-the-Box Research of Elaine Langer

In 1981, Harvard psychology professor Elaine Langer brought a group of men in their seventies to a location that was staged to give them the illusion that it was actually 1959. Everything was made to look like as though it was that year. Mirrors were removed, so the men could not see themselves. The vintage radio played Perry Como; on TV, the men watched the *Ed Sullivan Show*. They were told not to reminisce, but to act is if it was 1959. A control group was also brought to the same location, but those men were given no special treatment. Langer also made sure the men were treated as though they were twenty years younger. Before being told that they were in charge of bringing their suitcases upstairs, the men were tested on grip strength, physical dexterity, and flexibility, as well as hearing, vision, memory, and cognition. After a weekend time-warp get away, the men were stronger, more flexible, and taller. Even their vision had slightly improved. And those that witnessed the men leaving the retreat reported that they somehow appeared younger. Elaine Langer never published her research because she believed her unconventional study would have been rejected by journals, especially in 1981. "You have to appreciate, people weren't talking about mind-body medicine," she said. Yet her work has now become legendary. She has led many fascinating and groundbreaking studies in mindset, including one that compared adults in nursing homes. One group was given a houseplant to take care of, and told they would be in charge of their own schedule. The control group was told that staff would be taking care of their plants, and that they had no say in their daily schedules. A year and a half later, twice as many people in the plant caring group were alive. In 2010. A BBC TV show called *The Young Ones* did a remake on Langer's 1981 experiment with six aging British celebrities. She consulted on the project. Set in 1975, this group time-traveled to see shag carpets and kitschy art. The show aired in four episodes, and concluded with the six celebrities appearing remarkably revitalized. One even got rid of a wheelchair and swapped it for a cane. The show won a British Emmy. Jeffrey Redigar, MD, a professor at Harvard Medical School, said of Langer: "She's one of the people at Harvard who really gets it. That health and illness are much more rooted in our minds and hearts and how we experience ourselves in the world than our model even begins to understand."

THE TELOMERE EFFECT

Elizabeth Blackburn, PhD, and Elissa Epel, PhD, led a groundbreaking study on women, stress, and aging. Their study examined mothers who were caregivers to children with serious chronic health issues. The results painted a vivid picture of the connection between chronic stress and the length of their telomeres (a known marker of aging). The longer the moms had been caregiving, and therefore chronically stressed, the shorter their telomeres. In addition, if subjects perceived a greater level of stress, regardless of the actual stressor, the mothers' perception was related to the length of their telomeres. This deeply humanizing research carried out by Elizabeth Blackburn, PhD, and Elissa Epel, PhD, was also a part of their excellent book, *The Telomere Effect*. No one had ever done research on the chronically stressed, and especially on caregivers such as moms who had very ill or disabled children. The research, not surprisingly indicated a strong correlation between stress and aging. Blackburn and Epel discovered more: they found that some moms were more resilient to the chronic stress of caregiving. It seems that these parents had framed their reactions in a "challenge response," rather than a stress response. In a stress response, one feels hopeless. In a challenge response, the existing situation or condition is seen as a temporary setback. These mothers reacted with what is known as a challenge response and showed that people have the power to impact our telomeres even when under stress.

Another study looked at caregivers of relatives with dementia. Those caregivers that meditated for twelve minutes a day for two months, compared to a control group who did not meditate had a 43 percent boost in telomerase. "I have the power to impact my telomeres and I also have the power to impact yours," said the Nobel Prize-winning Blackburn. The power of the mind and our interconnectedness is part of the aging process.

Learning how we can skillfully harness our thoughts and perceptions on stress affects our health and how we age.

Many studies have shown that negative age stereotypes also have an adverse effect on health. Subliminal exposure to negative age stereotypes affect memory, handwriting skills, and gait. A 2016 study showed that older adults with "negative age stereotypes had greater loss in hippocampal volume and other higher predictive biomarkers for Alzheimer's." Another study showed that intervening and shifting negative age-related stereotypes to more positive stereotypes initiated a cascade of positive effects including improved physical function.

Dancing the Cha Cha

If it was that easy to be positive everyone would be doing it. If life is a dance, it is like the Cha Cha. Sometimes we take two steps forward and one step back. You can focus on the back steps, or any missteps, or stay intent on the dance itself. Sometimes in life things get "worse": you may miss a step, have a setback or illness, or lose someone you love. As in a dance, you could fall or accidentally trip our partners. Positivity is not about pretending that none of these things happened or not feeling the feelings around what happened. Positivity is about continuing to dance and looking for the good in each moment. It will be harder in life than in a dance, yet research and common sense suggest a resilient outlook will help you age well. I call it "seeing the world through mindful rose-colored glasses."

Rare Bird

American businesswoman, designer, and fashion icon Iris Apfel, ninety-six, also worked as a textile designer who specialized in historical restoration design projects including working at the White House under nine Presidents from Truman to Clinton. Age never, ever stopped her terrific sense of style and in 2005, the Costume Institute at The Metropolitan Museum of Art did a show about her, titled, "Rare Bird: The Irreverent Iris Apfel." A great success, the show made Iris a fashion icon at age eighty-four. When she turned ninety, MAC launched the Iris Apfel collection, "I am the oldest broad with a makeup line," she quipped. She has over 828,000 followers on Instagram, and she fights to proclaim a new paradigm of aging. "When they show ads about retiring, they always show these feeble people paddling canoes, playing golf, and jumping up and down on tennis courts. It's so ridiculous. There's lots of other things to do. You have to keep your mind active and get with it. And stay in the company of young people because they know what's going on, at least they think they do."

SCIENCE OF GRATITUDE

Many studies on gratitude have shown both the positive psychological and the physical benefits as well. Robert A. Emmons, from the University of California at Davis conducted a study on gratitude in which the participants were given the task of keeping a journal. They were divided into three groups: one that had to write five positive things that happened to them in the past week, another that had to write negative experiences and hassles that occurred to them, and a third which was told to journal any event that had a significant impact on them, without being told to focus on positive or negative circumstances. The group that journaled positive things that happened during the study was reportedly 25 percent happier than the other two groups, and reported fewer health problems. Another really important finding by Philip Watkins, a clinical psychologist at Eastern Washington University, found a correlation between depression and low gratitude levels. According to this study, clinically depressed patients showed 50 percent lower levels of gratitude than a control group. In his book, *Aging Well*, George Vaillant states that "those who have aged most successfully are those who worry less about cholesterol and waistlines, and more about gratitude and forgiveness."

Gratitude has been shown to balance heart rhythms and calm the nervous system. In a study with the HeartMath Institute and the US Postgraduate Naval School in California, gratitude was shown to increase levels of the anti-aging compound DHEA, a steroid produced by the adrenal glands.

Practice Tip

If you want to start practicing gratitude, begin by writing three things you are grateful for each day.

HELPFUL HUMOR

A sense of humor can help. When facing challenges, Super Agers tap into their amusement. Jean Calment, verified as the oldest living person, used to say, "I've only got one wrinkle, and I'm sitting on it." Humor can be a great go-to, when you are feeling low. One teenager from Ogimi, Okinawa, told the authors of *Ikigai* that she loved spending time with her great-grandmother, who was 103. When her great-grandma farted, she told her great-granddaughter that a loud train was passing by the house. The granddaughter said she liked to spend time with her great-grandma because she was fun and had a good sense of humor.

As we age, the brain begins to downsize, and if positivity has not been valued in the "save" part of the brain, the brain discards positivity. You can stop or slow down cognitive decline: see Chapter 11. Authors Hector Garcia and Francesc Miralles interviewed centenarians in the village where people live the longest and wrote down a few of the following quotes, which explain the long-lived villagers' mindset: "Don't worry," said one centenarian. "Live an unhurried life," prescribed another and simply, "Be

Optimistic." Having a slow, simple, and positive attitude towards life seems to be one of the secret ingredients to aging well.

TURNING 100 IS CAUSE FOR CELEBRATION AROUND THE GLOBE

Becoming a centenarian is an achievement recognized around the world. Find out how centenarians receive recognition around the world:

United Kingdom

In the United Kingdom, every centenarian receives a birthday card signed by the Queen herself, courtesy of the Department for Work and Pensions.

Japan

The Japanese government has a long-lasting tradition of gifting a *sakazuki* or silver cup to centenarians. Because the Japanese have the highest life expectancy in the world, the numbers of centenarians continue to rise dramatically, leaving government officials to look for a cheaper alternative. In 2009, the diameter of the sterling silver cup went from 4 inches to 3.5 inches. In 2016, the cups presented were no longer sterling silver, and instead were silver plate. Japan also holds a national public holiday, Respect for the Aged Day, on September 15. When you turn 100, you will receive a certificate from the Prime Minister on the first Respect for the Aged Day following your 100th birthday.

Barbados

In December of 2016, the country of Barbados issued a collection of stamps titled, Centenarians of Barbados. Twenty-seven centenarians were honored in this special tribute that coincided with fifty years of independence for Barbados. The stamps recognized the country's history of both triumph and suffering and tied it to the lives of centenarians who had directly experienced fifty years under British colonial rule and then fifty years of independence.

Philippines

A law passed in 2016 insured that Filipino centenarians receive 100,000 Filipino pesos (about $2,000) and are awarded a plaque. All Filipino centenarian citizens that live in the Philippines or abroad also receive a letter from the current President of the Philippines when turning 100. The first Sunday in October is National Day of Respect for Centenarians Day.

India

India bestows achievement awards for citizens over age sixty-five. Award categories include a general award for centenarians, and specific awards for sports, courage, iconic motherhood, and creative arts. Organizations who support older adults, and especially those that offer support services for older adults, such as housing and food are also awarded.

Ireland

People born in Ireland receive a nice surprise for their 100th birthday—2,540 Euros and a letter from the President of Ireland, wishing them a happy birthday and congratulating them on their longevity! Every year after you turn 100 you receive a specially designed coin that changes annually.

The United States

When you turn 100, expect a note from the First Family. And many people don't know that the White House sends birthday cards when you reach eighty (and to veterans turning seventy), and then they follow up at eighty-five, ninety, ninety-five, one hundred, and, every year after one hundred. What most people don't know is that you need to file a request for a card or do it for a loved one.

Similar traditions are in place in other countries, such as Canada and Australia. You must file a request to get a birthday signed card by the Prime Minister of Canada, and as for Australians, they get their birthday cards signed by the Her Majesty the Queen.

If you or a relative have a big birthday coming up, check with your own government for the latest birthday celebration procedures.

For a positive mindset as you age, take the reins of the mind and steer them towards the thoughts you want your brain to encode and remember. Your brain is like wet cement when you are a child. Then once you get past adolescence, "change is only permitted for those things that have captured the brain's attention, and only when the brain itself has judged those things to be beneficial." What this means is you are in control of what you deem important and savable by your brain. Dr. Michael Merzenich, known as the father of modern neuroplasticity, tells us that we must tell our brains what is important. You have the right to choose, not sit by idly waiting for good to come to you. Murali Nair, PhD, and Professor of Social Work at University of Southern California, studies centenarians around the world and notices a few common personality traits: "They always set goals. They say they are still young." Sometimes centenarians will have certain plans for the day or they will look ahead to a future goal such as taking their great-great-grandchild to their first day of school. Nair has studied and documented centenarians in China, India, Guatemala, Macau finds that most have a positive attitude and don't seem to be grumpy or sad.

Amazing and Inspirational

Irena Obera has mindset down. A retired teacher, she began her competitive running career a little later than most professionals, making nationals in 1959 when she was twenty-six years old. She ran in the 1960 and 1968 Olympic trials, and she found her stride when she became a pioneering master athlete. By the time she hit the forty-fives age group, wins and records became her norm, setting world records in the 200m in every age group from W45 to W70. IN July of 2014, she broke two records in the W80 for 80m hurdles and 200m hurdles. People who see her speed and agility are shocked to find out that she's eighty-four years old. "To me, I don't think of age as being a handicap. It's just a process. So why not live? Everybody tells me two things, "I'm so amazing and inspirational." I like the second part." When she was forty-one, she suffered a life set back when she was bedridden for a year after being diagnosed with sarcoidosis. After hearing about the first world masters championship to be held in 1975, she lay in bed, and made it a goal for her recovery just to make it to the event compete. She didn't come home with a medal that year, but it motivated her return. By the age of forty-five, she had become a dominant world force in track and field, smashing world records and winning world championships in multiple age brackets, W50, W60 and W75. In 2014, she became the oldest woman to break forty seconds in the 200m sprint.

FIRE OVER AIR

Modern culture could be described as out of balance. People are stressed and extremely busy. In the Blue Zone® books, Dan Buettner interviews nanogenerians and centenarians who live well balanced lives. Ayurveda describes age fifty and above as the Vata time of life, a time for inspiration, reflection, creativity, spirituality, and other qualities associated with air. Modern culture values power and dominance over wisdom. In Ayurveda, this could be described as valuing fire over air. One of the cultural issues that arises collectively and within each of us is the tendency to criticize and denigrate aging. It may be helpful to remember and realize that not all cultures put youth on a pedestal. Many cultures treat their grandparents, great-grandparents, and people over eighty as rock stars. A culture that values the fire stage of life of competition, aggression, and winning, instead of valuing the air stage of life, will also value drive and aggression over wisdom and inspiration. The point is that fire is not above air or below it. Fire is fire, and air is air. We need all elements for balance. When you embrace aging and cease to denigrate it, you esteem its qualities including wisdom, inspiration, and humility.

Logotherapy, developed by Victor Frankl, is a therapy concept based on life purpose. Frankl believed that life purpose helped one choose their attitude. Life purpose and attitude were central to Logotherapy. "Everything can be taken from a man, but one thing, the last of the human freedoms, to choose one's attitude in any given set of circumstances, to choose one's own way." wrote Victor Frankl in *Man's Search for Meaning*.

Singapore's Mother Teresa

One way to boost attitude is to volunteer. Helping others seems to boost mood and mindset like nothing else can. Teresa Hsu Chih was known as Singapore's "Mother Teresa." A social worker, yoga teacher, and nurse, she devoted her life to feeding and housing needy people, especially those in dire need, regardless of race or religion. "She's ninety-five, and she's looking after those younger than her. She doesn't care about herself. She only cares about others. This inspires me to follow her," said a certain Mr. Thanaraja, a volunteer at Teresa's nonprofit. Although she cared deeply for others, she had a simple, yet structured self-care routine. Born in 1898, she rose daily at 4 a.m. to do yoga, calisthenics, and meditation. She was a vegetarian who took up yoga in her sixty-ninth year. Known for her supremely optimistic spirit, she told people, "I prefer to laugh than to weep." Teresa Hsu Chih lived to the age of 113 years. Her organization, Heart to Heart (www.hearttoheartservice. org), continues to carry out her legacy of helping feed and house the poor in Singapore and beyond.

–PRACTICE PLAN–

Journal

Journal on resiliency. When and why do you give up? What triggers you to stop trying? Do you push yourself too hard? Will better self-care will help you to get through "the yuck?" Journal on seeing the bigger picture.

Express Gratitude

Daily Habits

Write down five things you are grateful for. Gratitude is one of the simplest and best ways to change your attitude.

Be Mindful

Take five minutes every day just to notice what you are thinking, seeing, feeling, smelling, and tasting. When we feel our senses, we step away from the mind. We step away from judgment. We become aware that we have the ability to choose our attitude towards our experiences. This knowledge of choice is a huge step forward.

Spice Up Your Life

Weekly Habits

- Exercise your "trying" muscles.
- Try something new every week; notice if you judge yourself or just feel good about trying.
- Develop resilience through trying. A Super Ager must continue to push through fear, worry, excitement, regret, and doubt. Try new activities or try to do something you have never done before every week.
- Write down your goals. Focus on your goals to sharpen your mindset.

Weekly/Monthly/Annual Habits

- Go to events that uplift your energy. If you aren't inspired, your mindset will suffer. When you are inspired, it changes your mindset.
- Here are some ideas for uplifting events:
  - Go to a concert or lecture.
  - Go to a museum.
  - Go see a movie by yourself or with a friend.
  - Get a massage or reiki healing.
  - Get acupuncture.
  - Walk in a park, forest, beach, desert, or some other place of natural beauty.
  - Have a party or meet friends for a drink.

Super Aging Habits

Daily Habits

- Compassion – Practice a daily self-compassion meditation (Chapter 11).
- Keep a gratitude journal.
- Make a God Box or a surrender box. If you find yourself constantly worrying or thinking about the negative, begin to write down your

negative thoughts and worries. Place these worries in a box. Place symbols of your worries in the box. If you find you cannot let go of your worries or negative thinking, allow yourself to indulge in thinking negative thoughts or let yourself worry, but put a time limit on it. Set your timer for fifteen minutes or even an hour. When time is up, put your thoughts back in the box. If it is too hard, try doing it the other way around, give yourself fifteen minutes or one hour worry-free, then let yourself worry like crazy the rest of the day or think negatively. You may find you like the worry-free time better.

- Stop Complaining – This is a fascinating exercise from the book, *A Complaint Free World: How to Stop Complaining and Start Enjoying the Life You Always Wanted* by Will Bowen. I was introduced to this book through yoga teacher Judith Lasater and her yoga club. She asked us to read it and try the exercise, which meant wearing a colorful soft plastic bracelet. The exercise went like this: each time I complained, I would have to move the bracelet from one wrist to the other. It made it oh so obvious just exactly how much I complained. Judith Lasater reminded us that it is human to complain. The real truth is that when we complain, we block ourselves from accepting things as they are or from taking action. Complaining creates a kind of inertia, a stagnation that quietly pollutes our mindset.

- Cease gossiping – Are you talking about someone else? Is what you are saying about another person something that you would feel comfortable saying to their face? If not, stop right now: you are gossiping. Mitch Horowitz, author of *The Miracle of A Definite Chief Aim and One Simple Idea: How Positive Thinking Reshaped Modern Life*, says that to stop gossiping is like taking a healthful pill. "This formula is free, and it can be yours immediately. It's only aftereffects are satisfaction, calm, and good spirits." Stop talking behind people's back to experience an immediate shift in mindset.

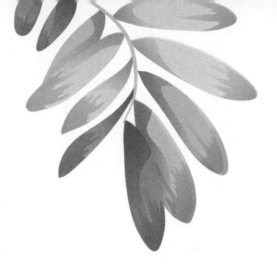

CHAPTER 4

You Are a Mosaic of Habits: Everyday Opportunities to Super Age

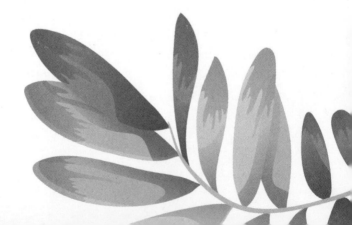

> ## *"Old age is like everything else. To make a success of it, you have to start young."*
>
> —Fred Astaire

Lifestyle makes up 75 percent or more of how you we age. You are a collection of your habits. Your habits are who you are. The biology of aging is extremely complicated, involving so many systems of the body, brain, and the nervous system. Not to mention that behavior can be complicated. What should you change, how can you change? It can seem overwhelming and impossible to change behavior. Yet if you can change one thing at a time, you can increase your confidence. Then you will realize you can change your habits slowly over time. You can make a big difference in your behavior with small, gradual changes. Super Agers cultivate healthy habits as an integral part of their aging plan.

If you're lucky, you started life with healthy habits that have continued throughout your life. The truth is not many in the western world begin life this way. Many who live in Blue Zone® areas won the habit lottery by being born into cultures that naturally integrated healthy aging habits. Don't worry if you didn't have healthy habits modeled around you by family and community: you are not alone. You can change your habits, and it is never too late!

There is no "typical" in aging; people age at vastly different rates. As humans increase in life expectancy and achieve better health through diet, lifestyle, and habits, there will probably be even more disparity in how people age. Many will increase their healthspan through good daily, weekly, and seasonal habits. There will be a steep increase in the numbers of outliers, known as Super Agers. The growing population of aging adults and our ability to remain healthy longer has made a mockery of previous stereotypes of aging. Even the World Health Organization has created a campaign to reduce outdated prejudices around aging, stating, "Ageism is everywhere, yet it is the most socially 'normalized' of any prejudice, and is not widely countered—like racism or sexism. These attitudes lead to the marginalization of older people within our communities and have negative impacts on their health and wellbeing." Human bodies are complex, with a myriad of diverse internal biological factors that influence our aging, as well as the external environmental and lifestyle factors that influence aging. Genetics is believed to account for 20–25 percent of the aging process, and the other up to 80 percent is in our hands. This book is about all of the relatively easy and inexpensive lifestyle changes that you can make to become a Super Ager.

Geroscience

This is an interdisciplinary field that aims to understand the biology of aging, age-related diseases, and quality of life, as well as other issues of aging. Geroscience spans multiple disciplines, including molecular biology, genetics, neuroscience, endocrinology, and genetics, among others. Traditionally, aging research focuses on single diseases and isolated conditions. Many scientific studies centered around aging fail because of the complexity of aging. "Geroscience" as a discipline was coined in 2007 by aging scientist, Gordon J. Lithgow of the Buck Institute for Research on Aging. Geroscience was recognized by the US Senate in 2010. "What has come out of our work is a keen understanding that the factors driving aging are highly intertwined and that in order to extend healthspan we need an integrated approach to health and disease with the understanding that biological systems change with age," according to former Buck Institute CEO Brian Kennedy. The

Buck Institute is "focused on the connection between normal aging and chronic disease," as well as extending the human health span.

Recoding

In 2014, Dr. Dale Bredesen of UCLA and the Buck Institute published the results of a small clinical trial on a multipronged protocol for treating Alzheimer's disease. The study scientifically demonstrated the possibility of the reversal of symptoms of Alzheimer's, a disease that is presently believed by western medicine to be irreversible. In his book, *The End of Alzheimer's*, Dr. Bredesen likens Alzheimer's to a leaky roof with thirty-six holes. The current medical model can't cure Alzheimer's because it only treats one cause at a time, which Dr. Bredesen likens to patching only one of the holes in the roof. If there are thirty-six holes, patching one of them will not do much good. The Bredesen Protocol, also known as ReCODE, is a collection of healthy lifestyle habits, combined with specific supplements that target biomarkers of Alzheimer's. By following the ReCODE protocol, you patch up many holes at the same time. Both the clinical trials that were published and Dr. Bredesen's continued work with Alzheimer's demonstrate that by patching even half of the "holes" in the Alzheimer's roof, symptoms can be reversed or arrested. Many declared Dr. Bredesen's protocol was "too complicated," or simply did not believe that it was possible to reverse or cease the progression of Alzheimer's in patients, yet the protocol is an oddly familiar set of healthy habits along with more complicated and specific supplements. The ReCODE protocol also divides Alzheimer's into three categories and uses specific protocols for each type of Alzheimer's.

The reason Dr. Dale Bredesen's work excites many health coaches, integrative doctors, and wellness professionals is because western science almost always focuses on one cause and effect and rarely, if ever, examines the effects of multiple lifestyle changes on chronic diseases such as Alzheimer's. There are many reasons that go into the one cause, one effect scientific model; all you must do is to take a look at the efficacy of Dr. Bredesen's comprehensive protocol to understand that this will be the future of medicine. Patients diagnosed with Alzheimer's can enroll in online support programs for Dr. Bredesen's protocol. In many degenerative diseases like Alzheimer's there are multiple holes in the roof. Using one drug is like patching one hole. And Alzheimer's is no different; if there are thirty-six different ways that brain health and physical health are degrading, you won't change much by patching up one hole with one drug or one therapy. Dr. Bredesen has found that he can reverse or stop the progression of Alzheimer's even by patching only half of the holes, so to speak. In a small trial of what Dr. Bredesen calls the ReCODE protocol, promising results were found for reversing or arresting the symptoms of Alzheimer's. Dr. Bredesen's ReCODE protocol gives hope for more mainstream adaptation of holistic lifestyle protocols for the treatment of Alzheimer's and many other degenerative diseases.

Bredesen Protocol, ReCODE:

- Optimize Diet
- Eat 3 hours before bedtime
- Eat during a 12-hour period and then fast for the other 12 hours
- Enhance autophagy (cellular clean up, especially in the brain) and ketosis (see Chapter 6)
- Meditate/Reduce Stress
- Optimize Sleep
- Exercise
- Optimize your microbiome
- Reduce Inflammation

START WITH SMALL STEPS

As a Yoga Health Coach, I am familiar with helping people to change habits gradually, as I will outline techniques in this chapter. It can take time and it is important to change gradually. I am trained in meeting people where they are and helping them to slowly transform their habits. When you change your habits, early success is important as it creates a momentum. Neuroscience affirms that the way to feel confident and cultivate success in habit change is to start small and build. I feel that this is the crux to changing and altering our habits, especially as we grow older. You start with small steps and things that are very easy to change, building to greater and greater levels of difficulty. Working at your own pace and building to more complicated habits or to habits that you may be resistant to ensures greater success.

As you read this book, you will be thinking about your own habits. You may read about something that does not appeal to you. Never worry about what you can't or are not ready to do. Ignore those habits that seem impossible or unappealing. Those are habits you can change later, or never. You are going for low-hanging fruit at first. As you realize the practice of Super Aging, I am imagining you will become emboldened and take on other small steps. Don't disregard the power of community. One of the biggest factors in healthy aging is strong support and community. Many of us in the western world don't have the traditional family ties and close knit communities that are a part of every Blue Zone® community. I predict that in the next thirty years, the human race will be rethinking communities. For now, begin to think about how you can look for support around you right now. Maybe you can read this book with a friend or start a book club. There's lots to read on aging, and you will be hearing about a lot more studies and advice about aging well in the next few decades.

Form Your Own Community to Support Your New Habits

Support can be critical to healthy habit change. Start with a buddy or a group. When you act in unison, the support becomes palpable. Suddenly changing long-ingrained habits becomes doable. Start a walking group, a volunteering committee, a healthy book club, or join a meetup focused on healthy habits or healthy aging.

Those that follow Dr. Bredesen's ReCODE protocol have an online support group for his complex protocol. Members of the group meet once a year and if it is their first time at the meeting, they are thrilled to meet online buddies in person. In my own experience as a Yoga Health Coach, my colleagues and I have found that creating support groups online or in person leads to far greater success in changing habits. The fact that our habits are part of our inner and outer ecosystem and are reinforced by friends and family can sometimes go unnoticed. When you feel supported in taking a step away from an old model of living, it can make change seem less overwhelming and scary. Have compassion for yourself as you transform.

It is never too late or too early to start your healing your lifestyle by embracing new habits that help you to feel good, look good and age well. When you feel isolated and alone, you will have more challenges in changing habits. Fear and apprehension can take over your mind when you lack support. Many of us live isolated lifestyles, so don't compare yourself to Some Super Agers who are a part of a culture that naturally supports Super Aging habits, like those who live in Blue Zone® regions. Some Super Agers have developed healthy aging habits at various stages of their lives, on their own, for many different reasons. It is possible to develop habits to find optimism in aging. Among all Super Agers, habits form the structure from which their purpose, dharma, or *ikigai* flourishes.

SCIENCE OF LIFE

I am a longtime student of Ayurveda, which considers daily habits to be integral. Ayurveda, meaning "science of life" in Sanskrit, codifies an optimal way of life, one that is in harmony with nature and the world. A person who lives in union with the here-and-now, who they are at the deepest level, and then in harmony with nature will live a long and happy life, according to Ayurveda.

"When I studied Ayurveda, yoga and enlightenment, I was told which habits I should be doing daily. Almost no attention was paid to behavioral science or how humans actually evolve their habits." observes Cate Stillman, in her book, *Body Thrive: Uplevel Your Body and Your Life with 10 Habits from Ayurveda and Yoga.* I resonate with this observation and wonder why behavioral science is not taught in every high school and college. Some acupuncturists, chiropractors, naturopaths, and MDs often don't instruct their clients in healthy habits and then almost never teach them how to set up a new habit using behavioral science. Cognitive Behavioral Therapists and other forms of behavioral therapists seem to be the only ones who are armed with the simple tools to identify, form, and then solidify healthy habits that benefit their clients. As the author of two books, I realized people liked to read my books on the Chakras and healing foods. They were inspiring, readers told me, but I wondered if anyone changed that much from reading them. On the other hand, books can make an impact when the author purposefully encourages habit change in the form of simple daily lifestyle practices that don't even take much time to perform.

When I joined the *Yogahealer* online community, I found myself able to integrate at least two habits that I had tried to change for at least a decade or so before meeting her. Cate Stillman and *Yogahealer* helped groups from all over the world shift their bedtimes, eat less meat, and to get up and get out and exercise. There is so much more to her habit-changing courses, and I, along with a team of editors and administrators, now run her health coaching blog at www.yogahealthcoaching.com.

One of the reasons I began studying Yoga Health Coaching with Cate resulted from a study that I worked on in 2010, when I was a yoga instructor for the PRYMS (Practicing Restorative Yoga for Metabolic Syndrome) study. This NIH-funded research study examined the effects of restorative yoga versus stretching in patients with Metabolic Syndrome, which is a cluster of symptoms that are an indicator that you are highly likely to get Type 2 diabetes. The lead researcher on the PRYSMS study, Dr. Alka Kanaya, gathered participants for our first class and orientation where she took some time to explain the study. This would be a year of restorative yoga for everyone and the study participants were required to engage in a home practice. As an instructor, I had to be sure my students were participating and do as much as I could to get everyone on board. During the orientation, Dr. Kanaya mentioned a previous study that she directed, *The Live Well, Be Well* study, which compared two groups. One group was waitlisted, while the other group received healthy lifestyle counseling, primarily by phone. After a year, many in the counseling group had made small, yet important reductions in risks for Type 2 diabetes. Why weren't interventions like this widely implemented, I wondered. As a yoga teacher, I felt I could make a significant difference in the lives of my students simply by counseling them on optimal health habits or setting up habits that I could ask them to perform. These initial thoughts led me to pursue "health coaching" as something valuable to offer as a health professional.

A simple phone call had such great benefits. What could similar health interventions do for yoga students? What if all we did was ask one question of our students per week about their health?

In studying Yoga Health Coaching, I learned about books and courses that explained the behavioral science and neuroscience behind habits. In yoga and holistic healing communities, many people rely on going to get help from a doctor or a practitioner. This works well when you are sick or not feeling well. However, there is much you can do to bolster health before you get ill. In Japan, preventative medicine is the model of care and it is no accident that the country has the highest life expectancy in the world. Preventative medicine or lifestyle medicine means integrating healthy daily and seasonal habits into your life. Understanding the connection between daily habits and preventative medicine deserves much more attention in western medicine and in many holistic practices. When you are sick, it is important to check with a doctor. However, cultivating healthy habits needs to be discussed more often by yoga teachers, acupuncturists, medical doctors, and the like. The assumption that change is too difficult for most people needs to change. Health coaches are trained to help people effectively change habits and enhance lifestyle choices for optimum health.

Body Thrive

Yoga Health Coaching was founded by Cate Stillman as a way to help yoga students and people interested in a holistic lifestyle optimize habits based on Ayurveda and yoga. She wrote the book *Body Thrive, Uplevel Your Body and Your Life with 10 Habits from Ayurveda and Yoga. Body Thrive*, which applies the most essential teachings of Ayurveda into a modern life by decoding the teachings into habits. Ayurveda is the perennial body-wisdom tradition that co-arose with yoga, the path of awakened living. The book describes a curriculum that every person can learn as a child, master as an adult, and refine as an elder for their body to thrive. The habits described in *Body Thrive* are simple and have been demonstrated to increase healthspan and lifespan, habits such as going to bed early, eating a hearty midday meal, exercising, eating more plants, and giving yourself regular oil massages, known as *abyhanga* in Sanskrit. To find a Yoga Health Coach to work with or for more information on Yoga Health Coaching visit https://yogahealthcoaching.com/find-a-coach/ to learn to put habits into place.

Twenty Years Younger

Jon Butcher, founder of multiple companies, including *Lifebook* and a Mindvalley Academy class, "Turn Your Life into a Living Masterpiece," credits daily habits and purpose with helping him and his wife to look twenty years younger than their biological age. "The key is the habits that you put in place and then being true to those habits. And the way that you are going to get that done is to have a strong purpose and that's what it always comes down to." Jon Butcher didn't set out to look twenty to thirty years younger than his age, yet his habits set him up for the life he leads today, teaching others in how to transform their health, have more joy, and have solid relationships, along with aging well. He gives classes at www.mindvalleyacademy.com.

HABIT GUIDELINES

Start small. Stanford behavioral scientist B. J. Fogg has branded the practice of starting new habits small as "tiny habits." Watch his popular YouTube video, "Tiny Habits." When we start small, we make change doable. We can use the small steps to create momentum. As a Yoga Health Coach, I have seen the opposite happen so often. People want big changes very quickly. They are so sick of their current situation; they want out immediately. Or sometimes it's the "Dream Big" syndrome gone horribly wrong. It's like creating a dramatic, bad break-up with their unhealthy habit. Instead, things can be much easier and healthier. And those sudden abrupt break-ups seem to almost always lead to the rebound effect. As the person finds that their big dramatic change doesn't work, it confirms negative thinking. Often the client decides to go back to the old relationship with their unhealthy habit. They seem to believe that they really can't change after all. I have seen this pattern of self-sabotage in myself and in others over and over. It is what has made me so committed to small, focused, doable, incremental changes.

Another habit-changing concept called kaizen comes from a Japanese word that means, "small, continuous improvements." Kaizen was adapted by Japanese businesses which needed to rebuild and restructure following the chaos and destruction that had occurred during World War II. Kaizen can be applied to habit change in thinking about the smallest tiny improvement that can be made. I have often noticed my health coaching clients wanting to change too much, too soon. This behavior creates a self-defeating loop. When a person wants to change a habit and then thinks about taking too big of a step in that shift, when it doesn't work, the person trying to change often gives up and believes that changing is futile. An example would be going to bed earlier. A futile step would be to try to change one's bedtime by one or two hours. While this may occasionally work for some people, most will fail and then give up. Instead of small steps, the person may consider the experiences as cement for their theory that they are a "night owl." Branding oneself a night owl instead of making smaller steps towards an earlier bedtime is not helpful. A kaizen step towards a new bedtime would be to set bedtime back fifteen minutes for an entire week, then increasing the earlier bedtime to thirty minutes earlier than the previous bedtime on the second week. In this scenario, it would take a month to shift bedtime by one hour. Kaizen has been proven over and over in studies, and I have seen it work as an effective and simple strategy in my coaching clients.

Habits and patterns are like roads that we have carved out in our life. The big habits may be like paved freeways, creating shortcuts or fast ways of doing things. Our habits may be useful and serve us in many ways. It's important to be able to objectify our habits. I like to think of my habits as roads. When a habit is brand new, it's like an off-road trail. I am walking or in an off-road vehicle. Change is scary. New territories are novel and intimidating. I am very present in my emotions on the new road. I may want to give up. Eventually, I cut a trail. Sometimes I pave it and make it real, as in, "I will do this every day for the rest of my life." Other times my habits may have been great superhighways in my twenties, thirties, or forties, yet as the years roll by, I realize that maybe I need to take a train or walk or dismantle that superhighway. Maybe the destination doesn't appeal to me anymore, or I don't need to go so fast. Maybe I can take a bullet train instead. I think you are getting it now. As we age, it is so easy to look back and be supercritical. Why did I do that for so many years? Or I have messed myself up? In this book, we are learning that we can cut new trails and pave new habitual roads. No looking back. No, rather, I mean: look back and appreciate the journey. After all, there have been people that have lived to be 100 who smoked, drank, and swore all their lives. There is no right way. There is only your way and the Wild West of the rest of your beautiful and precious life. Your life is a work of art. How will you live it?

Dinacharya

Dinacharya means "daily routine." In Ayurveda, synchronizing daily activities with daily cycles is one of the most important ways to support health. Western medicine has finally begun to understand the importance of the synchronization of human physiology with daily cycles, especially the rising and setting of the sun. Dinacharya includes activities such as waking time, elimination, hygiene, self-massage, bathing, meditation, study, work, and sleep.

Science has validated that within our brain, we have a master clock that regulates biological processes. Eating and sleeping at the wrong times can throw off this clock and cause chronodisruption. Other, secondary cellular clocks can be found in the liver, pancreas, and other organs. Chronodisruption or disconnection from the natural rhythms of daytime and nighttime has been linked to cognitive decline, diabetes, obesity, substance abuse, heart disease, and some cancers. In 2017, three researchers were awarded the Nobel Prize in Physiology or Medicine for understanding and explaining the role of circadian rhythm in health and in treating disease. *Scientific American* declared that circadian medicine "may revolutionize medicine as we know it."

Traditional Dinacharya

Morning:

- Wake before sunrise
- Scrape Tongue
- Brush Teeth / Wash Face
- Eliminate bowels
- Practice Yoga 15–30 minutes
- Shower/Bathe

Evening:

- Eat dinner early
- Meditate or practice gentle yoga
- Go to bed by 10 p.m.

Vata

As we grow old, we start to enter the *Vata* stage of life. Vata means air and ether combined. The Vata stage of life can be an inspiring, creative, and productive stage of life because life is about balance. Habits are grounding and earthy, and become more beneficial to our health as we age. As we age, we need habits more than ever. According to Ayurveda, habits contribute more to the energy of earth and provide stability that attracts healthy aging and creativity, joy.

According to Ayurveda, when we have a structure of daily and even seasonal habits, one can grow old with ease and grace. In many Super Ager cultures such as the village of Ogimi, healthy habits are an integral part of life and aging. If you don't belong to a community that supports habits, consider finding a health coach or group that will support you in healthy habit change.

–PRACTICE PLAN–

Familiarize yourself with habit change.

Read

- *Force of Habit* by Tasmin Astor, PhD
- *The Power of Habit* by Charles Duhig
- *The Miracle Morning* by Hal Elrod
- *Body Thrive, Uplevel Your Body and Your Life with 10 Habits from Yoga and Ayurveda*, by Cate Stillman
- *Mindset* by Carol Dweck
- *The Neuroscience of Change: A Compassion Based Program for Personal Transformation*, by Kelly McGonigal
- B. J Fogg's website, resources, classes, and tools on habit change at www.tinyhabits.com
- For Elise's courses on habit change, Super Aging, and Yoga Health Coaching, visit www.elisemariecollins.com

Daily Habits

Grab your journal and write about your own daily habits. Ask the following questions.

1. Do I like my habits?
2. What do I want to change?
3. What have been my past experiences with changing my habits?
4. How can I get really good at changing my own daily, weekly, and monthly habits?

Form a Healthy Habit Support Group

Cate Stillman has an outline for a book group to follow her book *Body Thrive*. Consider forming your own healthy habit meetup, book club, or group. You can meet at a local library, community center, or yoga studio. It doesn't have to cost money to change your habits, and finding a group is the single most powerful tool for habit change for those of us who have grown up in communities where healthy aging is not modeled by those around us.

Start Small

What habit do you want to change? Pick one, then take the smallest baby step: pick something that is so easy you can't possibly fail. Maybe you want to quit eating desserts. Your habit could be take one full inhale and exhale before you eat a dessert. Or your habit could be to begin exercising in the morning. Start with a walk around the block, or ten jumping jacks. Make it so easy you can't say no.

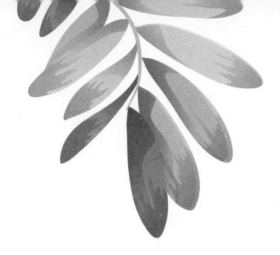

CHAPTER 5

Move Your Body to Slow Down Time

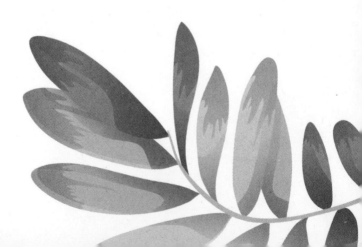

"Get up and do things, even if you don't feel like it. Sometimes you don't feel like doing this, that or the other. Do the thing that you don't like to do first, and get rid of it."

—Ida Keeling, 102, world recorder holder in 60m and the first woman to run 100m at age 100

Does your fitness routine need a boost of inspiration? Do you consider yourself too old to begin a new sport or workout routine? Consider Japanese centenarian Hidekichi Miyazaki, also known as "Golden Bolt," who took up competitive sprinting just after his ninetieth birthday. He now holds the world record for oldest to compete in the 100-meter dash, racing just a day after he turned 105. Do you feel like you have lost your edge? Do you fear you are over the hill? It is easy to internalize age-based stereotypes.

Exercise acts like a "superdrug" on the mind and body. Most doctors, trainers, and scientists will agree that not much can compare to the benefits of physical exercise. Aerobic exercise has been shown to decrease the risk of almost all types of age-related chronic disease. For the brain, nothing could be better than moving and strengthening the body. If there was one activity I would recommend to slow aging, it would be exercise. As a yoga instructor, I have seen firsthand the benefits of exercise on my own brain and body. I have also seen it transform my yoga students more than almost anything else. People that exercise change their bodies, and this ability to transform spills over into other areas of their life. Enduring the discomfort and the pain of strengthening, stretching, and endurance exercise to feel a payoff seems to be a lesson in Super Aging. Many who study the brains of Super Agers believe that a common quality of Super Agers is that they are able to push through the "yuck" part of learning something new. People that workout are all too familiar with pushing through the yuck. If you stop the moment a workout feels uncomfortable or a yoga pose hurts too much, you will lose many benefits. If you push through, you will learn that by practicing, by just showing up, you will reap the great rewards of pushing through the yuck. At the end of the day, once you have experienced pushing through, you know how you will feel better when you breathe, move, dance, run races, and do sit ups. Sometimes the yuck part is getting out the door or getting out the door. And it does not mean you are pushing yourself to overexertion.

You will feel better mentally, and you will feel better as you grow increasingly fit. You will be able to get out of bed at 6 a.m., or run to the finish line because you have learned and felt directly that pushing through has great benefits. The best way to grow the brain is to push through the discomfort, and the same goes for the body.

Artistic Visions

DeShun Wang never gave up on his artistic visions. As an actor and a model, he had some success. In his fifties, he took a risk and quit a job that guaranteed him a pension and security to further pursue his craft, creating an experimental mime performance he called "living theater." DeShun Wang didn't start hitting the gym until he was fifty years old and his, workouts seem to have fueled his career in later life. He says he only got serious about working out when he turned seventy. One day, he called his daughter on her cell phone when she was working as a designer for the Sheguang Hu fashion house. The designer saw her father's photo pop up on her smart phone screen—she shrieked and declared that this man must be in the upcoming fashion show. A few weeks later, DeShun Wang's famous catwalk was caught on camera. Expecting a dignified ballad to play during his final promenade, the speakers burst out a wild techno beat and DeShun Wang rose to the occasion, "I was on fire," he explained. Shirtless, exhibiting his incredible glossy ripped abs, flowing silver hair, beard and mustache, his explosive catwalk went viral. At age seventy-nine, he was an overnight sensation after his impromptu decisive circle on the stage was uploaded to YouTube. But he reminds us, "to prepare for that day I've been getting ready for sixty years." His brief sixty second prance lead to several feature film roles, a Reebok ad campaign, more modeling, and a documentary on his life story. Known as "the hot grandpa," DeShun Wang adds: "When you think it's too late, be careful you don't let that become your excuse for giving up." Now, at age eighty-two, he feels prepared for his newfound success as an international actor and model.

Exercise has been scientifically established as one of the biggest factors in healthy aging, especially for brain health, mental health and mood regulation. Exercise reduces the risk of almost every degenerative disease including, cancer, diabetes and heart disease. Studies on exercise and inflammation have shown that it decreases markers of inflammation and increases BDNF (Brain-derived neurotrophic factor), the neurotrophic factor that promotes growth and survival of brain cells. Exercise reduces symptoms of depression and helps with weight loss. And in the realm of slowing the aging process, some of the most convincing evidence of the miraculous benefits of aging come from research on the effects of exercise and telomere length.

Telomeres and Aging

What are telomeres, and why are they so important in the aging process? At the end of our DNA strands are protective, yet meaningless sequences of DNA that have been likened to the cap ends on shoelaces. Telomeres protect the integrity of our DNA but have no other purpose. When cells divide, part of the DNA sequence on the telomere doesn't get copied. Eventually, the telomeres wear away and the cells become dormant or senescent. These senescent cells are like rotten apples that turn other cells bad, or like hecklers at a theatrical play that begin to yell and disrupt the performance. Once cells become senescent, especially in aging bodies, they begin to ruin the show for other nearby cells, creating external effects of aging such as age spots and gray hair. Telomere length has a strong association with aging. The enzyme telomerase helps telomeres keep their length and sometimes grow longer if they have grown short.

Telomeres and Exercise

A 2015 study surveyed a large and diverse group of people on the extent of their exercise and the length of their telomeres. The study found that those who exercised more frequently and engaged in several different types of exercise had longer telomeres. Even more important to aging was the strong correlation between those participants who exercised less and the length of their shorter telomeres. In addition, middle-aged participants in the study (between ages forty to sixty-five) who were less physically active had the greatest prevalence of shorter telomeres, indicating that exercise in middle age seemed particularly important. A long-term study of British twins found that those that exercised moderately (less than two hours a week) had telomeres of someone five to six years younger, and that those that exercised for a minimum of three hours a week had telomeres of someone nine years younger.

In the past century, most of the western world has become increasingly sedentary. Perhaps in past eras of history, exercise would not have been as important, as physical activity was a natural part of living before twentieth century. In more traditional cultures, like most Blue Zones®, exercise is seamlessly woven into daily routine. In Okinawa, older adults walk, do household chores, and tend to their own gardens daily. Traditional homes in Okinawa don't have chairs or couches. Healthy nonagenarians and centenarians typically get up and down off the floor several dozen times a day, helping these elder Okinawans retain flexibility, agility, and tremendous lower-body strength. As a yoga teacher, I am aware that my aging students in the United States often have difficulty getting up and down off the floor, a requirement for the practice of restorative yoga. Moving from sitting on a tatami mat to standing up builds lower-body strength and balance, both of which essential physical attributes to healthy aging.

THE ORIGINAL BLUE ZONE®

The Barbaggio region of Sardinia was the original Blue Zone®. It is a mountainous region known for having the world's largest percentage of male centenarians. At first, researchers thought that a genetic anomaly accounted for the extremely high percentage of male centenarians in Sardinia until this theory was disproved. Dr. Gianni Pes explains that genetic markers of males in Sardinia do not differ much from the general population. Researchers now focus on lifestyle factors that accounts for the exceptional numbers of male centenarians in the villages of the Barbagia region of Sardinia to find the answers. The cardiovascular benefits of walking an average of five miles a day on steep terrain may be one of the answers. Sardinia is an extremely mountainous region unsuitable to farming, so almost all men are shepherds, which requires them to do the equivalent of a five mile Stairmaster challenge daily. Men also do a number of physically demanding jobs required by the family, the land, and animals they tend. On a typical day, a younger Sardinian male, Tonino Tola, age seventy-five, milks four cows, splits a half cord of wood, and walks four miles of mountainous terrain with his sheep before lunchtime. Now, that counts as exercise!

Why Blue Zone®?

Why is a Blue Zone® called a Blue Zone®? In 1999, Italian, Gianni Pes presented an epidemiological study of Sardinian centenarians at a conference on Experimental Gerontology. After hearing his presentation, Michel Poulain traveled to Sardinia, initially skeptical of the data which showed a great and disproportionate number of male centenarians in the Nuoro province of Sardinia. After verifying large numbers of male and female centenarians living in the region, Michel Poulain circled the area with a blue pen. The term Blue Zone® was later adopted to denote geographical regions that contained unusually high percentages of centenarians throughout the world.

THE BODY AS A TEMPLE

In Loma Linda, California, the only American Blue Zone®, local Seventh-day Adventists view the body as a temple. Adventists follow a vegetarian diet and abstain from smoking or drinking alcohol. Walking and going to the gym are part of a bigger picture of overall health that is part of the religious culture of Seventh-day Adventists. One of the religions founders, Ellen G. White, wrote about exercise in the nineteenth century, long before it was popular or scientifically validated for its health benefits. In *Healthy Living*, White stated: "God designed that the living machinery should be in daily activity. For in this activity or motion is its preserving power…. The more we exercise, the better will be the circulation of the blood." All other official Blue Zones® exist in remote areas or places often impenetrable to the stresses and unhealthy lifestyle woes that plague modern societies. Loma Linda's Blue Zone® circle came as a result of a collective group that upholds healthy behaviors together. Loma Linda demonstrates the possibility of communities coming together in cities, at community centers, and through common interests to create healthy lifestyle choices, including exercise, which will increase life expectancy of participants. This is something to note about this Blue Zone® that can benefit all people who feel troubled by the unhealthful habits of modern living. The Seventh-day Adventists demonstrate the power of a group valuing healthful habits, including exercise.

Moving our bodies in the modern world requires motivation. In all Blue Zones®, physical movement is woven into daily routine. Sometimes people are motivated socially to be active. Often being physically active is part of a job, as it is for the Sardinian shepherds. Because of the steep hills in the Blue Zones® of Sardinia, male shepherds have no need to join a gym. Okinawans in Ogimi all tend to their gardens. Some speak of gardening as their *ikigai* as well as a daily food supply. Because exercise has so many age-slowing benefits, making it a habit should be a top priority. What would motivate you to exercise? Would it help to have a buddy? One study in 2011 showed that people who held plank pose with a buddy held the pose for longer than those who held the pose alone. Would it help to join a class or have an accountability partner? Seventh-day Adventists exercise because it is part of their religious culture. How can you surround yourself by a culture or group that supports active living? Exercise is habitual to Loma Linda nonagenarians and centenarians. These Super Agers have a history of knowing and feeling the daily benefits as well as the accumulated effects of exercise. Skipping a day of exercise feels like not brushing your teeth to someone who has a strong habit. Think about how you can incorporate a strong daily habit of enjoyable exercise.

ENJOYABLE EXERCISE

If you want to start a new exercise habit, or just start exercising, find a fun movement based activity to participate in. If you do better in a group setting or you need more structure, join a class for dance, yoga, fencing, even gardening. If you want a group but maybe don't want the expense or structure of a class, join or start a hiking meetup, a runners group, or a boot camp posse. Whatever you do for exercise, make it pleasurable and doable, especially in the beginning when you want to make your habit stick. Engage in physical activities that bring you joy. This advice goes for exercise or any other ways we care for the body. Of course, when you are suffering from illness or health challenges, you may need to undergo treatments that are not fun! When you are well, take good care of yourself and enjoy that care. Exercise should be enjoyable and doable, or you will not do it.

One study demonstrated the importance of the right to choose exercise. Mice who had the ability to choose to run in a running wheel placed in their cage had higher rates of neurogenesis (growth of new brain cells) than mice who were forced to run. Another study published in the journal *Neurobiology of Stress* showed that mice forced to run in a treadmill had higher levels of stress hormones and neuronal damage to the hippocampus, the area of the brain that regulates emotion and organizes memory. While these were mice, it is highly likely this research would be applicable to humans. And when I think of my own history with exercise, feeling in control of my life and choosing the physical activities that I love or at least enjoy, especially with people I like (when applicable), greatly increases my compliance or daily practice of exercise. I have also found that making exercise and other self-care practices into habits makes a big difference. One way to implement a daily exercise habit is to do the same routine or yoga poses at the same time daily, even if it is only for five minutes.

DAILY PRACTICE

As a yoga teacher for twenty years, I know that my students struggle to create a daily practice. When one attends a yoga class or any fitness class, there are several things that make it easy to exercise. One is that there is an instructor telling you exactly what to do. You don't have to think or come up with a plan; planning and thinking about your exercise does take brain power and decision-making. If you are running your own business or you are a harried executive, you may not want to make any more decisions than you already need to. Psychologists refer to this as "decision fatigue." Perhaps you are "retired" and don't have that many decisions to make. Maybe you relish the idea of coming up with your own yoga sequence, CrossFit sequence, or boot camp routine. Some people are all-in for choreographing their workout. Others feel overwhelmed and may experience choice overload. I see this a lot for my yoga students and private clients. They ask me, "What should I do?" Either they cannot think of a yoga pose to do, or the choices seem overwhelming: there are so many poses. The same thing may come up with a myriad of different exercise or training techniques. This is where the *kaizen* technique comes in handy. You can refer to the more detailed explanation of kaizen in Chapter 4. Kaizen is the practice of taking a baby step, and it works so well for exercise and folding exercise into your daily routine. Let's say you want to start a daily yoga practice: here's what my advice would be. Start with three poses, for a more fit person, I may choose chair pose, downward-facing dog, and plank. For someone less flexible and fit, I would have them start in seated chair yoga poses, reaching their arms over their head and then touching the floor several times, twisting to one side and, if they feel up to it, getting in and out of a chair three to ten times. Pick a time of day. The time of day should work almost daily for you (weekends may be different). Remember, you are doing only three yoga poses, so no more than five minutes to start. Aim for consistency, not duration. Find a trigger for your habit. Daily triggers can include brushing your teeth, turning off your alarm, boiling water for tea, or making coffee. After the trigger action or event, next comes the habit in the form of an exercise sequence or workout. Next comes the very important finale: reward yourself. If your trigger is brushing your teeth, finish brushing and then you do your three poses. Maybe your trigger is an alarm on your phone, or after your cup of coffee. Then give yourself a reward: maybe going online for 5 minutes, doing a happy dance, or some other little thing you enjoy.

EXERCISE

Super Agers need to exercise effortlessly. How can you insert exercise into your daily life easily and effortlessly? Here are the top four areas you want to make sure that your exercise program covers: balance, endurance, strengthening, and endurance. There are also many different types of exercises you can do, such as yoga, tai chi, dance, walking, cycling, and rowing.

Good Form

Nanammal, age ninety-nine, of Tamil Nadu, India, has been practicing yoga since the age of three. "My grandparents worked in the fields and then would come home and do yoga on a mat. I joined them," she explains. She easily does *sirsasana* (headstand) and shoulder stand, yoga poses that many cannot do at any age. Following a traditional yoga routine, she rises at 5 a.m. to chant and greet the sun. She eats a simple vegetarian diet of greens, grains, and fruits. She shares her love of yoga with all of her children, grandchildren, and great-grandchildren, who all teach and help run the Ozone Yoga Studio in Tamil Nadu. In 1995, Nanammal traveled with her grandchildren to a yoga competition, only to see a participant disqualified for bad yoga form. She did not agree with the ruling and Nanammal took action. "I disagreed with the decision and went on stage to voice my opinion, only to be insulted by the judges as an old woman who did not know anything. Then I performed ten different yoga strokes (poses), including the 'peacock' and the headstand, right there on stage and received a standing ovation." Since that day, Nanammal decided to participate in yoga competitions and has made 250 first-place finishes in yoga competitions. Last year she was recognized on International Yoga Day in India, along with Tao Porchon-Lynch, as one of the two of the world's oldest yoga teachers.

Hatha Yoga

As a practice I have turned to for the past twenty-five years, I don't know how I would age without Hatha yoga. Yoga simply means union, and there are many types of yoga, including *Hatha yoga*. Hatha yoga is synonymous with "yoga" in the west, although in India and other parts of the world, yoga or union can be practiced in many ways: through meditation, service, chanting, pranayama (breathwork), concentration, and sense withdrawal. Because we are discussing exercise here, when I say yoga in this section of the book, I am talking about the physical practice of Hatha yoga.

Hatha yoga can build into so much more than just the poses and the physical benefits. As we age, we may want to slow down our sun salutes when a faster speed of practice no longer serves our needs. Longer sustained holds in yoga poses helps to ground the energy of Vata or air that increases as we age. Simplicity in our fitness routine may help as we age. We can use our yoga practice to look deep within as we strengthen our bodies, stretch tight muscles or fascia, and improve balance, proprioception, and agility.

You may be of the age that you can practice Vinyasa or "hot flow" yoga, but as you reach your eighth decade and beyond, you may want to rethink your practice. I am a huge fan of chair yoga because it can be challenging, yet accessible to all. I have taught chair yoga in many intergenerational settings, at an eightieth birthday party, a twentieth anniversary party, and for four generations of family. All can do the poses and those that can do more just do the same poses without holding onto a chair. Families and friends that do yoga together build trust and community.

Hatha yoga can be an excellent practice for your Super Ager Body. When you show up for those slower, deeper, more introspective poses, you can ask yourself a lot of evocative questions. What is irritating you? When do you want to escape? How is your breathing? Yoga poses done slowly and with introspection offer an excellent opportunity for internal growth. I believe this is union, the true meaning of yoga. The more I dig below the surface of my thoughts and the sensations of my physical body, the more I can begin to listen to and uncover my own deepest essence, what some would call my spirit. The "exercise" that one does while doing yoga asanas (poses) create flexibility, balance, strength, and elevated mood. Yoga is about connecting to something deeper within ourselves, and the physical benefits are icing on the cake. You can build balance, strength, and endurance with a good yoga practice. Many senior centers, community centers, gyms, and yoga studios have classes appropriate for all levels of students.

Chair Yoga

Chair Yoga can be a surprising way to stretch and practice building strength, agility, and balance. Anyone can do chair yoga, and it isn't just for older people. I love teaching intergenerational chair yoga classes. No one is afraid to try it, and you can use chairs to challenge younger people while allowing less-experienced yoga practitioners or older adults with no yoga experience to participate. Chair yoga is an excellent place to start at any age. When you learn to stretch and pose in a chair, you can literally take your yoga practice with you anywhere. Go to www.sunlightchairyoga.com

for chair yoga poses or chair yoga teacher trainings and to buy the book *Sunlight Chair Yoga for Everyone* by Stacie Dooreck.

Regain Your Balance

Some yoga asanas can help older adults keep their ability to balance or help them regain their balancing ability if it has deteriorated. Yoga helps develop the ability to feel where your body is in space; this sense is called proprioception. Practice balance in standing poses or on one leg in standing poses that require one leg to be lifted.

Endurance

Aerobic exercise improves circulation, has anti-inflammatory and antioxidant effects. Aerobic exercise reduces the level of a protein in the brain called BMP which slows the rate of neurogenesis and pauses the activity of neural stem cells. Aerobic exercise increases NOG (affectionately called "Noggin"), a protein that stimulates neurogenesis. Running has many brain benefits, and so does walking.

Hiit

High-Intensity Interval Training (HIIT) is known to burn fat, boost metabolism, and build muscle. Mayo Clinic researchers claim that it can also reverse signs of aging at a cellular level. "There's solid evidence that older, less active, overweight, and obese individuals can benefit from HIIT training," explains Dr. Edward R. Laskowski, MD, codirector of the Mayo Clinic Sports Medicine Center. "HIIT has also been shown to be very safe and effective in patients with heart disease and Type 2 diabetes. In all of these populations, HIIT programs can produce significant benefit for the cardiovascular system and improved metabolic parameters. And people seem to like it better than traditional endurance exercise." HIIT is a training technique where you give one-hundred-percent effort in quick bursts of exercise, such as sprinting for thirty seconds, and then resting and repeating.

HIIT elevates heart rate and burns more fat in less time, which gives this form of exercise an advantage over steady aerobic exercise.

In a study done by the Mayo Clinic, they compared HIIT, endurance, and combined training. All types of exercise showed good results (improving lean body mass and insulin sensitivity), but only the HIIT and combined training improved aerobic capacity and mitochondrial function for skeletal muscle. A decline in mitochondrial function is a common marker of aging in older adults. High-intensity interval training also improves a muscle protein content that enhances cellular energetic functions, as well as causing muscle enlargement, especially in older adults.

Strength

The aging process is associated with a decline in muscle mass and strength. Muscle strength is considered one of the biomarkers of physical capabilities as we age. Higher muscle strength helps us with accomplishing regular, everyday tasks, such as carrying groceries or climbing stairs. Engaging in a regular strength training program is able to reverse effects of aging on muscles.

Even more surprising were the results of a study that demonstrated that it is possible for those in their sixties to eighties to achieve muscle mass and strength improvements similar to twenty- or thirty-year-olds (who don't work out regularly) from a regular resistance training program. The older adults needed to do the extra strength training. When they lifted weights, they were able to achieve the muscle mass of someone fifty to sixty years younger. Strength training is also known to improve aerobic capacity, strengthen bones, decrease blood pressure, and stabilize blood sugar and blood cholesterol levels, as well as prevent and control heart disease and Type 2 diabetes.

Stretching Muscles

Yoga that includes stretching or an exercise program that includes stretching has many benefits. Stretching around the low back and hips can reduce lower-back pain. General stretching can improve posture and reduce the risks of falling. Stretching muscles make you less injury-prone and improves your mind-body connection as well as enhancing sports performance.

Radio Taiso

A gentle, all-ages warm up or exercise routine, Radio Taiso began in the United States in the 1920s, when Metropolitan Life Insurance Company introduced fifteen-minute radio calisthenics broadcasts as a way to promote better health. Japanese postal officials brought samples of the workout back home and the practice continues to be a popular regimented warm up almost a century later. The workout can last from three to ten minutes. Its catchy tune and movements work joints and muscles all over the body. Do it several times in a row, and it will be a workout. Find this simple upbeat daily routine by searching "Radio Taiso" in any language on YouTube.

-PRACTICE PLAN-

Rules of the Road and Mat for Super Ager Fitness

Try to build in at least one "never skip" daily habit: aim for consistency not duration. Then, when life gets hectic, you will never have to say, "I don't have time to exercise."

1. Find activities that you enjoy.
2. Look for buddies: someone to walk with, someone who will jog up that trail with you, someone to carpool with to the yoga studio.

Mix and match your routines and fitness companions. Moving in tandem makes time fly and entering the zone a no brainer.

3. Take a class. Sharpen your technique, learn new routines, feel inspired in your training. Do this when things start to feel stale or rote.

4. Remember the tiny habits adage, do one small thing until it grows. An apple tree starts from a seed, a fitness routine begins with a step. Start with a three-minute kitchen workout. Get up out of a chair ten times. Climb the stairs five times. What movement commitment can you make today? Choose something that you will be able to do every day because it is so ridiculously easy.

5. Use the Trigger–Habit–Reward cycle described in this chapter to develop daily practices.

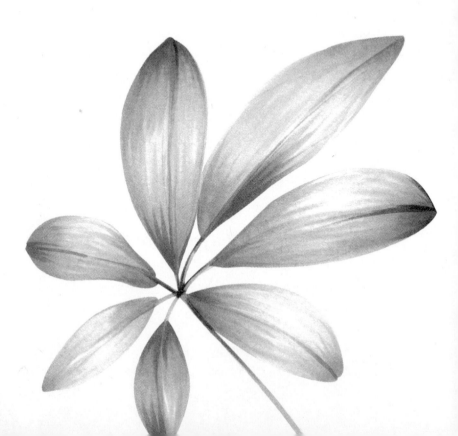

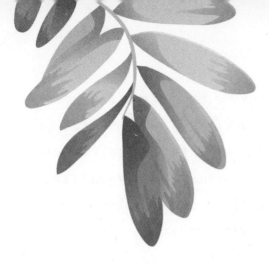

CHAPTER 6

You Are What You Eat, When You Eat, and How You Eat

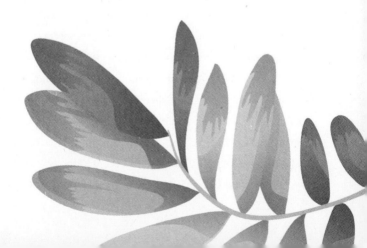

"If the Buddha came to dinner at your home, what would you serve? Fast food? A frozen meal quickly reheated in the microwave? Chances are you'd feed your honored guest a delicious meal prepared with love and care. But the next time you have dinner, what will you eat?"

—Hale Sofia Schatz, *If the Buddha Came to Dinner: How to Nourish Your Body to Awaken Your Spirit*

As the years roll by, food can be one of your best tools to postpone aging. We all have been reminded, "you are what you eat." This phrase conveys timeless wisdom. It's a meme, a truth from the Vedas, and a wisdom spoken by philosophers. It reminds us that we are made from what we put into our mouths. Yet the sum of the food ingredients that we put into our bodies is greater than the actual parts. We can look at food through the lens of nutritional science and we can also see food as something divine. Food can bring us balance and it can save us. Food has both sacred and mundane qualities. Food can have a dark side: we have to eat, but we can also use food to avoid painful emotions and spiritual truths. And food is not only about what you put in your mouth. Other important actions that are sometimes left out of the diet equation are how you eat, when you eat, why you eat, and who you eat with. These behaviors can be even more important than what you eat. A truly holistic approach to aging and food includes not only nutrition, but also the why, how, who, what of eating, as well as a sense of your own personal truths and wisdom around eating.

You may find that when you transform your relationship with food for the better, you discover greater freedom, wisdom, and creativity. In other words, when you eat well for yourself, you will undoubtedly experience healthy repercussions and very likely let go of other limiting beliefs that may affect your aging.

Fresh, whole foods that are nutrient-dense and prepared with love are considered light and enlightening in Ayurveda. Good food uplifts the spirit. While some foods may seem really "good," as in ice cream or a gooey donut, these foods may provide a temporary satisfaction and their quality is not as nourishing and sustainable. Yet at a celebration such as a birthday party, your anniversary, wedding, retirement, or special event, indulgent food can be an important part of ritual and celebration. If you have health issues that prevent you from eating certain foods, it is also important that you take care of yourself and respect your own boundaries. I want to stress that food is a form of self-love and self-care. Each day the menu may look different; yet if you keep in mind that your theme is to love yourself through nourishing yourself, you may find it easier to let go of some of your fear and self-criticism. If you are always eating the tempting addictive junk foods that surround us in the modern world, it eventually will catch up to you. At the same time, perfection, and rigid food guidelines would not be considered healthy. Flexibility, spontaneity, joy, and enjoying food with family and friends are an important part of eating. It's all about variety and context, and knowing your body.

As for the food itself, if your diet is not a whole-food, largely plant-based diet, you may want to consider making a change. Plants are the most nutrient-dense foods on the planet. The sacred quality of plants is that they capture the energy of the sun and the earth and the air. If that is too "woo woo" for you, remember that plants are power-packed with nutrition and fiber. Fiber helps you move food through your body and reduces spikes in blood sugar. If you are currently eating more of a meat-based diet or a ketogenic diet, there is more info below. Start small and slowly modify your diet by adding plant-based foods and trying recipes that inspire you. Nourishment includes calories, micronutrients, and the five Ayurveda elements. Food prepared with love has an intangible bonus ingredient. So, if you feel overwhelmed by the thought of changing your diet, you may want to skip changing anything about your diet right now or try something that sounds more enticing and doable for you, such as changing the time or times that you eat. Perhaps the best choice for you right now would be to cook more often or to allow yourself more time to enjoy a leisurely meal. Try not to get overwhelmed. Instead, find things that are doable and make small changes in your eating habits. Success begets success, and you will do better by starting small if you want to change or improve your own eating habits.

THE BREAKDOWN

How can you eat intentionally when there is so much conflicting information on how to eat, when to eat and what to eat? Let's break it down.

In a scientific model, food is the building material that our cells need to generate and regenerate healthy tissue, bones, blood, and organs. "Other than genes, it is hard to think of something that can be more powerful than food in determining whether someone is going to be 100 or die before fifty years old," says Valter Longo, Professor at the USC School of Gerontology and head of the school's Longevity Institute. The science behind nutrition, what to eat, when to eat, and how to eat has great value and can inform a holistic model of eating and food. Food is a very personal choice and your relationship to food can be complicated and multilayered. If you have eating habits that you want to change or update, read this chapter carefully and look for ways to update and give yourself a nourishment makeover.

Dosha (Also Known as Prakriti)

Each person is unique and has their own blueprint. Like a snowflake or a fingerprint, you have a dosha that is unique only to you. Your dosha is a combination is usually a combination of two or three doshas. Your dosha can be a guide to precision or personalized medicine.

Here is a brief description of the three doshas:

- **Pitta**: People dominated by the Pitta dosha are fiery and intense. Pitta types like to win or get it right. When they are out of balance, they are hot-headed, angry, or irritable.
- *Vata*: Those with more of the Vata dosha are creative, delicate, and dreamy. Sometimes Vata types run out of steam. When a Vata is out of balance, they may be called a space cadet, or lose important items such as wallet, jacket, or keys.
- **Kapha**: The ultimate nurturer, Kapha types are slow to move, steady, and have incredible stamina. Kaphas love connection and in relationships. A Kapha type will be told, "You are my rock," by those that love them. When out of balance, Kapha people will have trouble getting off the couch or getting out of bed.

To find your dosha, try one of these recommended online quizzes:

- https://www.banyanbotanicals.com/info/prakriti-quiz/
- https://theprimeclub.com/dosha-quiz-intro/
- http://www.mapi.com/doshas/dosha-test/index.html

BLUEPRINTS

In Ayurveda, each person has a unique blueprint or mind-body-spirit type that can guide their healthy choices in life. This mind-body-spirit type can also help guide food choices. So, according to Ayurveda, there is no one-size-fits-all guide to eating. Instead, take yourself to the Super Aging buffet, where there are lots of healthy choices. How you fill your plate with food is your choice: it's personal and it's for you. And according to Ayurveda, your food life may be more about when you decide to eat or how you eat. Maybe your Super Ager strategy is to cook for yourself and your family more often. There is research and ancient wisdom and many choices. Make the food choices that serve you, your family, and your lifestyle best. Eat consciously!

Covergirl

At the age of sixty-nine, Maye Musk inspired women around the world when she became the world's oldest Covergirl in 2017. She tweeted, "Thank you to everyone who has complimented me on my @COVERGIRL ad. After fifty years of pounding the pavement, I have achieved what many models wish for. #atlonglast #almost70 #dontgiveup #workhard." Some dreams may not come true when we are eighteen, twenty-five, or thirty-five: Super Agers don't let age get in the way of dreams; they keep on dreaming. One of the ways Musk supplemented her income during her modeling career was by advising others on what to eat. A registered dietitian with two master's degrees, Maye quips, "I'm a nutrition scientist who models." Her never-surrender attitude landed her features in a Virgin America ad campaign, a James Bond video game and a Beyoncé video. Her commitment to nutrition sustained her as she continually broke barriers in a business that often abandons older women. Maye prefers a hearty breakfast of whole-grain bread and eggs to avoid mid-morning hunger and the blind eating that follows. For lunch, she takes a big salad with farmer's market veggies and some protein. She cooks a mean fifteen-bean soup for dinner, adding ample vegetables in a big pot, freezing extra for lunch and another dinner. She snacks on fresh apples and grapes to satisfy sweet cravings. She's nixed the gluten-free trend and goes for a general diet focused on superfoods such as pumpkins, sweet potatoes, spinach, greens, and cruciferous veggies such as broccoli and cauliflower. "First of all, the skin is the largest organ in the body, so if you're going to eat well for your heart or for your kidneys, or for your liver, then pretty much that will help your skin as well." She's also a mom to three adults, well known as scientists, entrepreneurs and rule breakers: Elon, Kimbal, and Tosca.

EATING FOR STABILITY

In Ayurveda philosophy, you have a unique blueprint, and accordingly that personal prototype informs your diet, how you exercise, and many other lifestyle choices. In essence, your diet should fit who you are and support your own life and aging process. In general, because you are in the air stage of life when you age, the cornerstone of healthy eating in Ayurveda at this stage is found in choosing warm, nutritious whole foods to support stability and steadiness. There are many foods and ways of eating that have age-slowing benefits. Researchers often come up with conflicting reports on the best foods to eat, when to eat as well as how to eat. Not everyone wants to admit that there are many healthy ways to eat and that each one of us is unique. The trick is to find the plan that works for you. In this chapter, you can look at which foods and strategies fit your mold. Next you can evolve your diet gradually and make adjustments along the way. If you are in it for the long haul as a Super Ager eater, be kind to yourself and take things slowly. If you already rock your daily menus with foods that balance you and help you feel great, then consider yourself a Super Ager eater. If you would like to steer your eating to a little healthier ground, try one small change at a time. After the first habit sticks, you can move on to the next small change. Before you know it, you will have made big strides, even when the original change seemed overwhelming. Many of the suggestions in this chapter come from Ayurveda, others from research and common sense. This may mean gradually shifting to a more plant-based diet for one person. It may mean adjusting to eating less at night for another person. For you, the first change could be adding fresh and dried spices to your foods. There are so many ways to optimize healthy eating for aging. And as you have noticed, there is no one-size-fits-all. This chapter will fill you with new ideas and new ways of tweaking your meals and healthy eating plans. The most important Super Aging diet is to feed yourself in a way that lets you love yourself. For some this might mean occasional ice cream, for others, a strict ketogenic diet. Read on for inspiration.

Consuming more plants and eating whole, unprocessed foods translates to eating in harmony with nature. Some centenarians eat wheat, meat, dairy, and sweets. What works for one person may not work for another. In Ayurveda, moderation is key, as well as listening to your own inner guidance. Many Super Agers follow a stringent eating plan, while others seem carefree. When we think about food as something that supports our life and brings us joy, it takes off some of the pressure. In Ayurveda, food supports and infers intelligence. No food is inherently bad or good. The quality of what you eat becomes the quality of your body and tissue. And what you eat is also metaphorically what you see in your newsfeed, on the highway, in the movie theater. You eat words, experiences, and relationships. In other words, if you are stressed by what is happening in your life, it will affect your digestion.

Food itself has qualities of intelligence, lightness, or even heaviness or lethargy. A donut might temporarily make you feel lazy and foggy. But that same donut shared in joy with a grandchild could be a longevity elixir. When you eat to balance your mind, body, and spirit, you make adjustments along the way. You may find it helpful to think of food as a way to support your emotions and worldly endeavors. Generally whole, fresh, unprocessed foods give you a light and expansive feeling.

Precision Medicine and Personalized Eating

In western medicine, there is a trend towards personalized, precision medicine. "One size fits many" is no longer the only option, for several reasons. The costs of many kinds of lab tests have decreased dramatically in the last few decades, making it easier to formulate individualized health guidelines; moreover, the costs of guesswork in variable diagnosis for medical doctors is becoming cost prohibitive. With the rise of Big Data, technology can provide more personalized healthcare solutions. But personalized, precision medicine has always been the mode of treatment in Ayurveda, Traditional Chinese Medicine (TCM), Functional Medicine, and several other forms of traditionally based healing systems. If you are not sure what to eat or how to eat, seek the advice of an Ayurvedic Physician, Functional Medicine Practitioner, Licensed Acupuncturist or nutritionist who can help you develop an individualized eating plan.

HOW, WHY, AND WHEN OF EATING

The food we consume comes in the context of our lives. A beautiful and colorful stir-fry with homegrown vegetables and spices prepared with love for a happy family has vibrancy and intrinsic intelligence. The food we enjoy should complement and support our lives. The act of sharing meals with loved ones can be a more powerful health booster than "perfect" nutrition.

Do not ever forget the "how" to eat, "why" to eat, "who" we eat with and "when" to eat. Those are all up at the top of the list with the "what" for us Super Agers. You are shifting paradigms in order for your consciousness to permeate the entire "eating experience."

The cycle of hunger and satiation is as old as humankind. Some of our collective disconnect may be because people have lost touch with nature or because we have an abundance of food and aren't starving anymore. It is important to enjoy the feeling of hunger and then the satiation of a meal deliciously prepared with love, eaten alone or with friends. Digestion is part of the fire element, and it is considered important to feel hungry in Ayurveda because it demonstrates that digestive fire is present and ready to transform and assimilate food.

In Ayurveda, the most viable way to heal the body is to repair or balance our digestion. Interestingly, here is another area of health that it seems that western medicine is either just catching up or validating what the Ayurvedic sages have spoken of for thousands of years. The gut rules all. Our microbiome and digestion greatly contribute to optimum health. If your digestion seems to be lacking in any way, a personalized consultation maybe helpful. For specific health and digestive issues, always consult a medical doctor, Functional Medicine doctor, Ayurveda doctor or practitioner, Naturopathic doctor, or licensed acupuncturist. If your digestive system needs an overhaul, try doing a seasonal cleanse or microbiome makeover.

Agni

Agni means fire in Sanskrit, and in Ayurveda it refers to digestive power. If you have low agni, consequently your digestion becomes weak and food is not properly transformed. Food that is not converted to energy and cellular tissue becomes cellular waste. Indeed, this is aging, the accumulation of cellular waste. According to Ayurveda, one of the ways we can slow aging is by keeping our agni burning strong. Think of your agni like a wood-burning stove. If you have built that fire with kindling and paper, it will have the ability to burn a log. Strong digestion has the same properties as a strong wood-burning stove; you can eat anything. If you don't have as strong digestion, you may not have as much freedom in your diet. And in this metaphor, when it is time to sleep, you let the fire die down so that the body can use the agni for other purposes besides digesting food. You would not go to bed and leave your wood-burning stove burning at full capacity. The good news is just like that wood-burning stove, you can take steps to carefully kindle your digestive fire. Probiotics or a gentle cleanser, like triphala, are a few ways to kindle the digestive fire. There are so many ways to get your digestive fire burning strong. Find an Ayurveda professional at www.ayurvedanam.org or a Yoga Health Coach at www.yogahealthcoaching.com.

LIFESTYLE ADAPTATIONS

A small pilot study demonstrated that changes in diet, exercise, stress management, and social support affect the length of telomeres for the better. The lifestyle interventions that participants undertook were similar to lifestyle recommendations called for in Ayurveda. One group made the following changes: they ate a plant-based diet, walked thirty minutes a day, practiced yoga, performed breathing exercises, completed daily meditation, and attended a weekly support group. When compared to a control group who made none of the aforementioned lifestyle changes, those that made the broad range of changes experienced a significant increase in telomere length, and that increase was correlated with how much the participants adhered to the recommended lifestyle adaptations. Those that followed a plan that included yoga, a vegetarian diet, meditation, and breathing exercises had longer telomeres and increased telomerase activity, demonstrating the longevity effect of a yogic lifestyle.

Consistent meal times can be a significant and often overlooked strategy to aging well. Often people concentrate on the "what" to eat, with little consideration to the "when." Ayurveda and many ancient systems have always emphasized the rhythms of the day and stressed the importance of dependable meal times. Parents often put their children on schedules because the value of a steady schedule for young children seems innate to being human. Yet somehow, modernization has pulled many humans away from this idea that consistent meal times have importance for the body. Western medicine has made significant breakthroughs in the emerging field of circadian medicine. There is more of a movement to restore the balance of a more standard schedule of sleeping and eating as research continues to point to its importance. The science on circadian rhythm continues to confirm the health value of eating at consistent scheduled times as well as establishing the damaging effects of unsynchronized feeding and sleeping. Ayurveda has long recommended that you eat on a regular daily schedule.

Your body is growing less consistent and your body needs consistency to age well. Our meals need to be at around the same time every day, almost every day. Consistent mealtimes support digestion as we grow old and enter the air stage of life. Life is blowing in the wind; we need everything to be as solid as possible, this includes our meals. I recall my grandmother, who lived to be ninety-five, eating regular meals. She was pre-diabetic, as long as I can remember. She never took any medication for her condition, but always kept her blood sugar in check with consistent, regular meals. On the other hand, my immediate family and our daily meals were all over the place. The message I got growing up was to value studying, learning, and work over regular meals. I still believe in the value of learning and work, but I now realize that regular meals support our intellectual and career pursuits, not undermine them. I recognize the incredible value that my grandmother's regimented meal routines gave to me. My mom was a working mom who had a career in the 1970s. Our family ate late. My mom loved to cook, yet our meals were often erratic and usually late. The food was always amazing, since my mom was always a foodie before the word was even invented.

I learned about good, healthy whole food, from my mom, but not food schedules: then, my grandma helped as I saw how her meal plans and times helped her outlive her husband by twenty-plus years. Later, when I studied Ayurveda, I saw the value of my grandma's routines, even though her food could barely touch the amazing food my mom produced in the gourmet kitchen I grew up in.

Health Should Be Your First Priority

Bernando LaPallo died peacefully at age 114 on December 19, 2015. He saw Babe Ruth and Lou Gehrig play baseball. When he was 112, he was recognized at Yankee Stadium for being the team's oldest living fan. His father, a Brazilian doctor, brought him to the United States when he was only five years old. He told Bernando, "Your health should be your first priority." Bernando drank a cup of cinnamon tea and sipped daily superfood smoothies. In his "youth," Bernando LaPallo worked as a five-star chef on cruise ships. Shipmates teased him and called "the rabbit eater," for his diet of raw foods. "They're all dead now," Bernando said of those who taunted him. He took up a new career in his 70s, practicing massage, herbalism, reflexology, and holistic podiatry in Queens, New York. In his late nineties he became a longevity speaker and later an author. Fortunately, Bernando left a legacy, revealing countless health tips on his website, numerous YouTube videos and his book, *Age Less, Live More*. Bernando ate at the same time daily, finishing his first meal before 5 p.m. most nights. He walked a mile and half every day, using a walker only when the weather was bad. He had a deep faith in God and drank mocktails when he socialized with friends: orange juice and soda, garnished with a cherry and an orange slice. He ate blueberries and cantaloupe, and soaked his grains and legumes before preparation; he loved making black beans and rice as well as a special barley soup. He was very proud of his skin, which he rubbed daily with olive oil. "Nothing hanging," he would say. He ate fish a few times a week, never consumed dairy, and enjoyed broccoli, asparagus, kale, collard greens, nuts, and seeds regularly. "Cleanliness is next to Godliness," Bernando affirmed, "keep your colon clean."

COOKING

A study of 1,888 Taiwanese men and women over the age of sixty-five found that those that cooked five days a week or more were 47 percent more likely to be alive after ten years. The study's lead author, Mark Wahlqvist, stated, "It has become clear that cooking is a healthy behavior. It deserves a place in the lifelong education, public policy, urban planning and household economics." Ayurveda considers the preparation of food as a sacred act and one of utmost importance. Caring for yourself by cooking for yourself and your loved ones has benefits beyond the science of healthy eating. The cooking study interviewed participants on various lifestyle factors including asking questions about all of the activities required for meal preparation. "The pathways to health that food provides are not limited to its nutrients or components, but extend to each step in the food chain, from its production, to purchase, preparation and eating, especially with others," added Wahlqvist. Researchers in the study came to similar conclusions that can be found in Vedic texts. Preparing food has multidimensional benefits for mind, body, brain, and spirit. Cooking in this sense is synonymous with preparation; it doesn't necessarily mean heating food, but it can mean that. When you mix, cook, prepare, and fabricate your own meals, there is a special ownership, creativity, and alchemy that may be difficult to scientifically quantify. Common sense, the aforementioned research, and Ayurveda recognize the health building power of making your own meals.

Preparing food for yourself and loved ones promotes health and wellbeing. The more you infuse your own energy into food for yourself and your family, the more healing the foods will be. A secondary boost is that cooking is a good brain exercise. When you cook, you utilize your senses, sight, touch, smell, and taste. When you try new recipes or try to remember recipes from the past, you stimulate the brain and memory.

Cooking and Recipe Tips:

1. Go to the library. Check out cookbooks that appeal to you. Try recipes and different styles of cooking. Buy only the cookbooks that you are certain you will use regularly.

2. Look for recipes or food blogs online that inspire you. Try your favorite recipes from cooking and bloggers. Or just search for recipes you want to prepare, and then adapt recipes according to need and taste.

3. Subscribe to a meal kit plan. Although meal kits have definite drawbacks such as utilizing lots of unnecessary packaging, meal kits provide a level of ease for those that feel overwhelmed cooking or by trying to make fresh food at home. By scaffolding the process of meal preparation, you avoid the shopping or the stress of forgetting critical ingredients. Younger and older adults may feel more adventurous trying out new recipes and cooking techniques. Meal kits can foster confidence and be a baby step towards more adventurous cooking.

MEAL PLANNING

Planning meals is one of the best ways to reduce calories, eat healthier food, reduce calories, and avoid making unhealthy choices because you are starving and have nothing planned for dinner. Avoid fast food and other temptations by planning your meals a day, a few days, or a week in advance. If you are comfortable with technology, meal-planning apps can really be of service in organizing recipes, offering suggestions, and even auto-populating shopping lists. If you prefer old school meal planning, create your own meal-planning spreadsheet. You can find a plethora of premade hardcopy meal-planning sheets by Googling or searching on Pinterest for printable meal-planning sheets. Most of them are good for the week, and it may be good to have a copy on display. If you have a multigenerational home of kids, teens, parents, and grandparents, family members will love to know what's on the menu in advance. If it is just you or you and your spouse or partner, there are still multiple benefits to advance planning. A 2017 study showed that even ravens plan their meals ahead of time, so why not you? With the pen and paper method, you can stimulate neurons by holding a pen and writing, something shown to be good for your brain. Extra points if you draw or decorate your meal plan. For Super Aging, following a daily meal routine is the first critical habit to put into place. Planning meals can make regular meal times doable. Apps such as Yummly, Paprika, Pepperplate, and Meal Plan can help organize your meals, recipes and shopping in the digital domain.

Eat Big at Lunch

Most important meal, drum roll please…have your biggest meal of the day for lunch. Yes, I said lunch. Why lunch you may wonder? Well, truth be told, in Ayurveda this is your biggest meal of the day. It is also a time when it is easier on your body to indulge and combine foods that might not digest as well together. Lunch as the biggest meal of the day when the sun is highest in the sky and your body produces the most bile (which breaks down fats). Your agni is strong at lunch, and your body can digest more food and a greater variety of foods. It seems that we have collectively forgotten to eat a big meal midday. During the Industrial Revolution, people went off to work and wanted to share a big meal with family in the evening. Now people are either doing the same thing, or are just in the habit of eating a big meal at dinner. The issue though is that the biggest meal of the day needs the most digestive fire and that digestive fire is strongest around noon and in the window between 10–2 each day.

You can have fun going out for lunch, cooking a big meal for lunch, or just eating lots of food at a time between 10–2 p.m. by yourself. Digestive fire and bile is most productive and strong between 10–2 p.m. In Ayurveda digestive fire or agni aligns with the sun. When the sun is high in the sky and it is the warmest time of the day is the best time to eat your biggest meal. If this is not currently in your Super Aging habit repertoire, then you can gradually build in this habit. You will be creating a structure that will yield a great payoff in terms of long-term greater health and energy. Our habitual or haphazard meal times and meal spacing are considered of utmost importance for Super Ager. Interestingly, most Blue Zone® nanogenarians and centenarians have consistent meal times.

Spacing, Stacking, and Snacking

Practice meal spacing not meal stacking. Cut the snacking, especially mindless snacking. Eat only when you are hungry. Eat three meals a day, and on rare occasions have a small snack. As you age, you won't need to eat as much so even two meals can do the trick. Ayurveda has always recommended giving digestion a break between meals.

In Blue Zones®, such as Sardinia, Italy, Ogimi, Okinawa, and on the Nicoya Peninsula in Guatemala, adults eat at set times and never snack.

Keep a regular schedule of breakfast, lunch, and dinner and avoid snacking. Allowing your body to rest between meals rather than grazing or snacking will actually stabilize blood sugar. Some nutritionists used to recommend six small meals a day for optimal blood sugar. Research has demonstrated that snacking or eating small meals actually has a detrimental effect on glucose levels. So, nix the between-meal tapas and enjoy more food at mealtimes.

Eat a Light Dinner

Supper used to be called supper because it was a light meal that supplemented lunch as the largest meal of the day. It is a fact that in most of the Blue Zone® habits include eating a light evening meal. Nicoyans eat two breakfasts and a light dinner. Larger lunches are habitual for Ikarians and Sardinians. Okinawans don't do dinner. Even in English, the word "supper" actually meant you were supplementing the biggest meal of the day lunch with a little soup or leftovers to get you through so you would sleep and go until breakfast. American nutritionist Adelle Davis was known for her demonstrative quote: "Eat breakfast like a king, lunch like a prince, and dinner like a pauper." If you are accustomed to eating a big meal at dinner, take your time changing up this habit. It may take time, months or even years, to break the habit of eating a lot for dinner. Take your time; you will have plenty of time to change this habit. If you already eat a light dinner, you know the benefits. If not, you will eventually feel the benefits of a light evening meal, keep the pounds away, and sleep better with less in your belly later. You may find it difficult to eat less at night, when family and friends insist on late meals and nights out on the town. It is not part of mainstream habits, but I have found it is easy to live this way even when friends and family don't agree with my plans.

Flip It at Dinner

So, if you are eating your biggest meal of the day for lunch, what do you eat for dinner? The simple answer is to flip it: eat dinner for lunch and lunch for dinner. I would avoid heavy food at dinner (especially meat and cheese, or whatever heavier foods that your body tolerates), and lean on those foods for lunch instead. Have dessert with lunch. Also remember to check with your digestion periodically. One of the hallmarks of aging is that your body is changing so keep checking in and noticing how your body feels, how your digestion is going, and how your elimination is. If all is well, full steam ahead. If not, it may mean time for a body evaluation. Time to reevaluate and recalculate.

How to Recalibrate or Recalculate as You Age

Sometimes you will need to evaluate your body and sometimes your mind as you age. Your digestion slows down, or you may experience a personal crisis. Perhaps you are taking care of an ill family member. Life is filled with unexpected stresses. Make room for constant check-ins; they will keep you healthier and adjusting as you age, not recoiling or losing confidence. Use crisis or trauma as a time for heightened self-care and awareness. It may be a time to throw out all your healthy eating guidelines and simply pray and meditate. Or at another time you may feel as though it is best to double down on good food and sleep. As you age, you will need to take good care of yourself. Your mental, spiritual and physical health as you age is always a moving target, so don't ever be afraid to recalculate what you need or recalibrate your self-care. Consult your medical doctor, Functional Medicine practitioner, naturopath or Ayurveda practitioner if you need more support.

INTERMITTENT FASTING OR TIME-RESTRICTED FEEDING

Caloric restriction profoundly affects the pathways and biomarkers of aging. Scientists have searched for ways to mimic caloric restriction, and have found that Intermittent Fasting or Time-Restricted Feeding has remarkably effects to caloric restriction. Because caloric restriction so clearly extends lifespan, intermittent fasting has been embraced by many as the next best thing. Before meal stacking, Ayurveda always, always emphasized meal spacing, which is a form of intermittent fasting. Ayurvedic meal spacing naturally evolves into a form of intermittent fasting, where there is a 12–16 hour feeding gap between dinner and breakfast. Ancient wisdom called for people to give their digestion a break between meals. Modern study of intermittent fasting has concluded the same thing. Intermittent fasting can also be called Time-Restricted Feeding, or TRF, referring to the window of time when eating takes place. Look at testimonials for how intermittent fasting works (good and bad), by searching for TRF on the Internet. To be clear, there are a few ways to do intermittent fasting and there are many ways this "diet" has been named.

Let's look at the science and the reality of what intermittent fasting does to the body. Intermittent fasting promotes ketosis. Intermittent fasting has also been called Time-Restricted Feeding, or TRF. For twelve hours of TRF, you could eat your last meal at 9 p.m. and then eat breakfast at 9 a.m. If you wanted to go for a longer fast, skip breakfast. Ayurveda recommends eating your last meal by six o'clock or around the time of sunset. If you are eating over the course of eight hours a day, you would have sixteen hours of fasting. That would be a Time-Restricted Feeding or TRF period of eight hours a day. If you eat over the course of twelve hours a day, that would be a Time-Restricted Feeding or TRF period of twelve hours a day. Dr. Dale Bredesen describes his Alzheimer-reversing protocol as "Keto-Flex 12–3." The "12" means that you are doing Time-Restricted Feeding for twelve hours of eating and then twelve hours of fasting. The three in "12–3" refers to eating three hours before going to bed. Time-Restricted Feeding and Intermittent Fasting are the same thing.

Some researchers and scientists believe that Time-Restricted Feeding will not be as triggering a description to the general population because the word fasting is not a part of the definition. In any case, this style of eating has been practiced for thousands of years in Ayurveda and has been extensively studied in recent years. Research has confirmed that eating during a window of 12–16 hours will help stabilize metabolism. In addition, eating an earlier dinner will help your body digest and metabolize food before sleeping, further supporting healthy metabolism and digestion. These habits are considered critical by many anti-aging experts and Ayurveda specialists. Valter Longo, biogerontologist and director of the Longevity Institute at the USC Leonard Davis School of Gerontology, says, "It turns out that it is important to stick very close to twelve hours of feeding and twelve hours of fasting." He calls this a periodic diet, which mimics the dramatic age-slowing benefits of calorie restriction without any of the risks and extreme discomfort. Not all intermittent fasting programs or protocols recommend eating earlier at night; however many Blue Zone® cultures and centenarians eat early, light dinners. Lighter dinners could include soups, salads, steamed veggies with oil and spice blends, rice and lightly sautéed vegetables, and maybe a little meat or fruit.

Eating on Vacation

When one is on vacation or at a conference, don't sweat it. Go off of your light, early dinner; change the plan. When I took a family trip to Italy this year, many restaurants did not open until 8 p.m. If I was traveling by myself, I could skip dinner and fast between a late lunch and breakfast. Instead I traveled with three generations of family. I ate lunch and dinner and skipped breakfast. This way I did temporarily tax my digestion by having a heavier meal at dinner, but I continued to practice intermittent fasting by skipping breakfast and allowing my body to process the heavier Italian food that I enjoyed. Consider changing your meal plan on vacation to make it easy on yourself if you practice, Time-Restricted Feeding or Intermittent Fasting. You may want to skip breakfast if you have a late dinner or maybe you will stick to a light dinner. Do what works for you.

Intermittent fasting also has brain benefits. It increases BDNF which promotes neurogenesis and reduces overall neural inflammation. Once again, Ayurveda has always recommended meal spacing or the practice of not eating between meals to give the digestive system a break. Intermittent fasting has become popular in the past few years because of the mounting scientific evidence that intermittent fasting can give you the benefits of calorie restriction, yet without having to reduce food or nutrients. Ayurveda has always stressed that one should meal space, rather than stacking. Meal Stacking, which means eating many small meals, was promoted in the past few decades as a way to combat low blood sugar, yet this way of eating does not allow the body to clean up and digest food. The digestive system never gets a break.

Ketogenic Diet

A ketogenic diet is a low-carb, high fat, high protein diet. Foods that are high in carbs produce glucose and insulin, while a keto diet basically produces ketones in the liver, which are later used by our bodies as energy. Ketones are produced when the body uses fat for fuel.

The benefits of a ketogenic diet are numerous: weight loss, lower blood sugar levels, increased mental performance, energy, better skin, etc. Ketosis takes place when the body lacks carbohydrates to produce glucose, and the body goes into fat burning mode and produces ketones instead. When blood level ketones rise to a certain point, you are in ketosis. It is a complex process that switches the body into a fat burning mode. People have been using ketogenic diet for almost 100 years for some health conditions, such as epilepsy. Only in the past five to ten years has this diet become extremely popular. It is very therapeutic for people who have insulin resistance issues because a ketogenic diet reduces blood sugar levels, which helps in lowering glycation levels. If not kept in check, high glycation levels impart tissue damage, escalate diabetic complications, and cause aging-related cellular damage.

A ketogenic diet slows the aging process in several ways. One is by reducing oxidative damage that happens when extra oxygen radicals are produced in cells which, in return, exceed antioxidant capacity. A ketogenic diet reduces cellular damage associated with aging by increasing uric acid and other antioxidants in the body. A ketogenic diet has a positive effect on a number of neurological disorders, especially on Alzheimer's and Parkinson's disease. A study done by John C. Newman and Eric Verdin showed that a ketogenic diet increased the lifespan, healthspan, and memory of aging mice. Mitochondria produce energy in our cells which impacts our longevity. Dysfunctional mitochondria are a biomarker of aging. Research on ketosis has demonstrated beneficial effects of the diet on the functions of mitochondria. A ketogenic diet has been shown to increases the neurogenesis in the hippocampus. Also worthy of mentioning is that being in ketosis increases mitochondrial glutathione, an antioxidant that works directly within the mitochondria, which is important because antioxidants that we acquire through food don't make it into the mitochondria easily.

A keto diet is also beneficial because it decreases inflammation in the body. Low-carb diets in general decrease a number of triglycerides, which are known as the fatty acids. Elevated triglycerides are indicators of heart disease risk and inflammation.

Autophagy

Autophagy comes from the Greek roots auto, meaning "self," and phagein, meaning "to eat": autophagy literally means to eat oneself. Autophagy is kind of cellular cleaning of old, worn-out cellular debris. In autophagy, junk cell materials are repurposed into new cellular materials. Autophagy is highly regulated because it is a destructive mechanism in the body. Eating turns off autophagy and fasting turns it on. As we age, autophagy becomes less effective and our bodies and cells have lots of cellular waste that accumulates. Many scientists believe that this cellular gunk is one of the causes of aging and that maybe the excess gunk that builds up may be one of the causes of disease. One scientist even called this process garbaging.

Super Ager Constipation Cures

Constipation occurs more frequently as we age. Our cycles of digestion and elimination are of utmost importance in Ayurveda. When you keep digestion in balance, health follows, according to Ayurveda. If your digestion is backed up, then we cannot properly assimilate and absorb the critical nutrients that help as we age. Note that there is no clear medical definition of constipation or chronic constipation. Constipation is broadly defined as an unsatisfactory defecation characterized by infrequent stools, difficult stool passage, or both. Ayurveda would agree more with Emile Gautier, who said, "Freedom of the bowels is the most precious, perhaps even the most essential of all freedoms, one without which little else can be accomplished." And by the code of Ayurveda, you should poop every morning, with infrequent exceptions. If you need to heal your gut, so to speak, you may need to consult one of the following for more in depth and personalized treatments: Ayurveda practitioner, naturopath, licensed acupuncturist, health coach, or medical doctor. Always contact your doctor if you are temporarily constipated. Use the following list of foods to help with proper elimination.

"Eat Baked beets, stewed raisins or apples" Cate Stillman, author of *Body Thrive* and founder of Yogahealer.com Cate is known for her no nonsense and down to earth approach to helping people changing their health habits and find simple solutions to everyday health issues. If you recently cut out coffee or tea it will take time for your body to readjust its natural urges, so up your intake of fiber and or foods that stimulate elimination:

- Take Castor Oil: 15–60ml on an empty stomach or with food (will work more slowly if taken with food.) In 2–6 hours you should be eliminating.
- Psyllium powder is good for diarrhea and constipation. Psyllium comes from *Plantago ovata*, an herb from India that contains both soluble and insoluble fiber. Psyllium husks bind to partially digested food that's passing through the stomach to the small intestines. Psyllium husks have been found to soften stools and increase elimination, especially in adults who are chronically constipated. Take 1–3 tsps. with water when constipated or for regular elimination.
- Take banyan botanical triphala tablets, or prepare triphala tea, 1 teaspoon per 8–10 ounces of water.
- Calms magnesium powder can also help. Magnesium initiates peristalsis, so taking magnesium supplements, or the Calms powder mixed with warm or hot water or juice, can help with regularity.
- Up your greens intake or drink green juice to stimulate elimination.
- Rub your belly with Castor Oil, do it on both sides of the belly button.
- Do a warm oil massage on your belly and then add a heating pad.
- Add fresh aloe to your morning: drink-2-3 ounces.
- Add chia seeds to your smoothie or make chia pudding: use almond milk or coconut milk and mix with chia seeds, add fruit to garnish.
- Eat fermented foods, look in Sandor Katz's book *Wild Fermentation* for good recipes or buy fermented foods at your local supermarket or health food store.

PLANT-BASED DIET

Nondenatured, whole foods are at the crux of any healthy eating plan, especially as we age. Eating simple whole foods and a plant-based diet can be surprisingly delicious and easy. A plant-based diet refers to focusing on eating plants, which are nutrient-dense and fiber-rich. There are many shortcuts to preparing fresh, whole foods. According to Cate Stillman, "Unlike most diets, a plant-based diet is defined by what it focuses on, not what it excludes. You maximize consumption of nutrient-dense plant food." A plant-based diet is all about the plants crowding out other, less-desirable foods such as processed foods, unhealthy fats, oils, and excess meat consumption (or any meat at all). Like all changes, you can gradually ease into eating more plants. Later in this chapter, we will go over specific foods that are wonderful for aging. The details make us think we need to spend hours upon hours in the kitchen preparing special meals, but this is not true. When we start from the big picture, the details seem to fall easily into place. The big picture helps us to fall back into faith and a feeling that we can do this. When you feel confident, then you can fill in the specific food details, depending on what is on our agenda for the day, for the season, or the time of life.

EAT LOCALLY AND SEASONALLY

Prepare seasonal and local foods. It will be tastier, more nutritious, and less expensive. Local, seasonal foods hit a home run every time. Get in touch with the food that is produced within 200 miles of where you live and what is growing abundantly near you. You will thrive on many levels. I recommend going to farmer's markets weekly or at least monthly for the experience of seeing the food that is seasonal and local. And when you go to a farmer's market, you can talk to farmers about the food. Ask a farmer or farmer's market vendor how different produce was grown. Ask about recipes or other preparation tips. Another possibility is to subscribe to a Community Sustained Agriculture (CSA) box. These boxes will give you a variety of fresh fruits and vegetables. Lots can be gained by subscribing to a CSA box. The value that comes from knowing what grows well locally and in season will help you with your food choices and will often help your budget and your waistline. If you have a garden, a small plot of land, or containers, you can grow your own vegetables, fruits, and herbs. In the Blue Zone® of Ogimi, Okinawa almost all of the older adults up to age 100 tend their own vegetable gardens. Gardening is good exercise. It is also relaxing and pleasurable to spend time in nature. And the best benefit is that you will grow wonderful nutritious food. Note that a ketogenic diet can be vegan.

SPICES ARE THE VARIETY OF LIFE

Spices can add so much to each and every meal. We can use common fresh spices such as parsley, basil, cilantro, rosemary, or oregano. One small, yet powerful dietary change that you could begin today would be to add spices to every meal. Spices are extremely nutrient-dense and most, if not all, spices have tremendous anti-aging and healing properties. If it feels too overwhelming to change your dinner or lunch or eat more plants, try this one small thing: sprinkle dried spices such as turmeric, cumin, or oregano on your food. Or you chop up fresh cilantro or parsley and sprinkle it on your beans or veggies.

Super Agers supplement their diet with medicinal plants that support health. Herbs can be eaten fresh, made into teas or tisanes, taken as tinctures, or eaten in dried form. There are many ways to take in medicinal and culinary herbs. Super Agers may drink herbal teas or mix dried herbs or tinctures into juices, teas or smoothies. Liquid medicines will be assimilated by the body more easily than pills in most cases, especially by older adults.

CULINARY HERBS AS MEDICINE

Note that just because we use herbs in cooking does not mean that these herbs are less medicinal than strictly medicinal herbs. Use fresh or dried herbs to boost digestion and add powerful Super Aging properties to all of your meals. The good news is that your food will taste better too! Here is a list of powerful herbs for aging:

- **Basil**: an antimicrobial, with a powerful punch of antioxidants. Use basil to reduce inflammation and prevent infections.
- **Parsley**: high in vitamin C, chlorophyll, and antioxidants.
- **Fennel**: a nutrient-rich herb that calms digestion, especially intestinal spasms. Fennel is good for menopausal women, as it contains phyto-estrogens that have a natural hormone balancing effect.
- **Fenugreek**: can help keep blood sugar levels stable and has estrogenic qualities, making it good for menopausal women.
- **Garlic**: is antibacterial, antimicrobial, and antiviral, and may help lower blood pressure. Sulfur compounds in garlic are responsible for its medicinal properties.
- **Dill**: acts a backup to boost antioxidants in the body and is used medicinally to treat depression. Dill also has antimicrobial properties.
- **Ginger**: helps with digestion, is good for everyone according to Ayurveda, and reduces inflammation, especially that associated with rheumatoid arthritis. Ginger is also a natural blood thinner and decongestant.
- **Turmeric**: contains curcumin, which is a potent anti-inflammatory agent. One of the biggest culprits of age-related damage is inflammation. Turmeric guards against Alzheimer's and helps the liver detoxify from carcinogenic chemicals. It has heart protective benefits and anti-cancer compounds. Put a shaker of turmeric on your table and use it daily!
- **Cardamom**: is a carminative (flatulence-reducing) herb with antimicrobial properties and detoxifies the body. It is a good for asthma and improves

circulation. Cardamom can boost your mood by reducing symptoms of depression.

- **Cinnamon**: helps with digestion, helps control blood glucose levels, and has antioxidant and anti-inflammatory properties.
- **Nutmeg**: contains a feel-good phytochemical that made it very expensive in the 1600s. It helps induce sleep and contains phytochemicals such as myristicin and macelignam, which have been shown to boost brain health.
- **Cumin**: aids digestion and is a carminitive spice. It also helps decrease symptoms of asthma, bronchitis, and insomnia. It is nutrient-dense and helps with circulation. Animals fed cumin seeds showed a strong decline in blood sugar or hypoglycemia, a condition that leads to diabetes. Cumin also helps rev up circulation in the body.
- **Cilantro** (fresh) & **Coriander** (dried): can chelate heavy metals and detoxify the body. Cilantro has antioxidant properties it reduces anxiety, controls blood sugar, and keeps your urinary tract healthy. A study published in *Molecular Neurobiology* found that diets high in turmeric, pepper, clove, ginger, garlic, cinnamon, and coriander helped to reduce inflammation associated with neurodegenerative diseases such as Parkinson's, MS, and Alzheimer's.
- **Cayenne**: clears phlegm in the upper respiratory tract. Cayenne actually cools the body, and can help ulcers feel better because it kills bacteria that cause ulcers and then helps to rebuild cells in the stomach and intestinal walls. Cayenne is also a potent antioxidant.

HARA HACHI BU

Remember the Okinawan saying that means eat until you are 80 percent full. This is called *Hara Hachi Bu*. If you like to eat until you are full, try this: eat to your heart's content between 10 and 2 p.m. Eat whatever you want (eat dessert!), but eat only one meal in this four-hour period. According to Ayurveda, your digestive fire or agni is highest at this time. Think of a wood-burning stove. You just get it started in the morning, using kindling, cardboard, and newspaper; by ten in the morning, it is burning strong, the logs are red or white hot, and you may add a log or two until two p.m., when you start to slow the fire down. By evening the fire is dwindling. If you eat a lot of different foods or overeat, the best time to do that would be at lunch or brunch, when that fire consumes all. Otherwise, follow the Hara Hachi Bu, 80 percent full feeling for breakfast and dinner. Chances are you are going to realize how much better you feel when you don't stuff yourself, especially at dinner. If you feel you can only follow Hara Hachi Bu, try dinner, as that is the most important meal to start reducing. If your typical dinner makes you feel 100 percent full, try reducing to only 95 percent and then move slowly to 80 percent.

If you get hungry late at night or must work late, try to have soup, miso soup, or a snack of a spoonful or two of honey. Soup has the quality of water, so it feels filling and moves down. The element of water is close to earth, which makes us feel heavy and grounded when we feel anxious and light. Try soup or honey on nights when it feels impossible to fast through the night. Or eat a few spoonfuls of honey or a bowl of soup if you get hungry before bed.

SUPER AGER FOODS

- Colorful fruits and vegetables – Phytonutrients in fruits and vegetables are healing compounds that support the health of the brain, the body, the organs, the skin, and the heart. Blueberries, for example, have powerful anthocyanins.
- Foods that contain NMN – Nicotinamide mononucleotide (NMD) is a precursor for Nicotinamide adenine dinucleotide (NAD), which

can be found in every cell of the body. NMN can be found in broccoli, broccoli sprouts, cabbage, cucumber, edamame, avocado, and tomato.

- Foods that contain NAD – NAD can be found in small amounts in the following foods: whole milk (use raw or whole milk if possible), peas, and asparagus. NAD is found in every cell of the body and has many age-reversing properties, such as enhancing mitochondria, increasing cognitive function, and metabolism. It mimics fasting because it mimics the actions of sirtuins produced during fasting. Low levels of NAD also interfere with DNA repair. Research is being done on the age-slowing effects of NAD molecules on the body.

- Rich wild greens – Rich wild greens are a big part of the Ikarian, Okinawan, and Sardinian diets. Greens have especially high amounts of chlorophyll and other healing and detoxifying nutrients.

- Berries –Blueberries, raspberries, blackberries, and strawberries are extremely high in antioxidants.

- Protein – Beans, nuts, seeds, whey powder, spirulina, yogurt, eggs are good sources of protein.

- Fiber-rich foods – Foods such as lentils, okras, Brussels sprouts, and any legumes contain fiber, which is quite beneficial.

Fiber

A 2016 study published in the journals *Gerontology* surprised researchers it revealed that a person's fiber intake was the greatest indicator of "successful aging." Fiber intake was more important than total carbohydrate intake, glycemic index, sugar intake, and an individual's glycemic load. The study followed 1,600 adults over fifty and considered those who stayed disease-free and healthy "successful agers." Participants who ate 29 grams of fiber were 80 percent more likely to live a longer and healthier life. All fiber is plant-based, so a "plant-based diet" is the easiest and most simple way to increase fiber intake. The top fiber foods include avocado, green peas, lentils, raspberries, almonds, sweet potatoes and edamame. You can also supplement your diet with fiber by adding ground psyllium husks, ground flax seeds, or chia seeds to soft foods like soups, teas, smoothies, yogurt, or any liquid. Let plants be the foundation of your diet, and a low fiber intake will never be an issue.

Two Types of Fiber

- Soluble fiber – This kind of fiber absorbs water and becomes like a gel. It bulks up in your digestive system, giving a sense of fullness as an added benefit. Soluble fiber acts like a sponge, clearing out the digestive system.
- Insoluble fiber – Found in whole grains, vegetables, and fruit skins. Because this type of fiber doesn't break down, it ferments and supports good gut bacteria. It also acts like a broom sweeping through the colon to clear out undigested foods and toxins.

Healthy Fats

Ayurveda has always been pro healthy fats. Here are some healthy fats that should be incorporated into your diet:

- Avocados, avocado oils
- Butter
- Ghee / clarified butter
- Coconut oil
- Extra Virgin Olive Oil – For Extra Virgin Olive Oil or EVOO, be aware that many less expensive brands are not purely olive oil and often contain chemicals and filler oils. It is worth it to buy high quality EVOO. It's a powerful antioxidant and anti-cancer oil, often used in Mediterranean diets. Don't use EVOO to cook at high temperatures.
- Fish oil – Your body can not produce Omega-3 oils, so you must get it from a dietary source such as fish oil or flax oil.

- Flaxseed oil – Flaxseed oil is a great vegetarian source of omega 3 oils. The body will convert Flax oil into omega 3 oils.
- Nuts and seeds
- Nut and seed oils such as sesame oil, walnut oil, borage oil or evening primrose oil and other above-mentioned oils.

Anti-Inflammatory Foods

Inflammation is one of the biggest culprits in the aging process. If we are healing from illness, have chronic inflammation or just want to reduce any inflammation in the body. Increase the following foods:

- Ginger – Add this spice powder to drinks, vegetables, and any savory dish for additional flavor. Use fresh ginger by peeling and then finely chopping the ginger. Sauté the ginger in ghee or coconut oil for 30–60 seconds and then add it to your food, or add vegetables and sauté.
- Tart cherry juice or tart cherry
- Black Strap Molasses with baking soda
- Fresh Vegetables, fruits, nuts
- Root Vegetables – All roots have a calming effect and are good foods for many reasons for aging. Roots come from the earth and therefore give those that eat them a calming, grounding quality.
- Beets – Beets are very potent age-slowing vegetables, rich in vitamins and minerals, they are good for digestion and heart health. Beets are known in many cultures as an aphrodisiac that helps increase your sex drive as you age.
- Daikon

Aging can cause changes in the microbiome. In particular, levels of bifidobacteria are high in the body when we are young but decrease with age. Bifidobacteria reduce inflammation and helps you to absorb nutrients. Some probiotic foods that can help you boost this microbiome-boosting bacteria are brine-cured olives, apple cider vinegar, yogurt, kefir, tempeh and miso.

Water

As one ages, the thirst area in the brain decreases. Unfortunately, even as your desire for water decreases, hydrating becomes increasingly important as you age. More than ever as you age, the habit of drinking water is important. I can't emphasize enough that making drinking water a habit is important. This means drink it first thing in the morning every day without fail. Ayurveda recommends drinking warm water with lemon. Do this every day, just like you brush your teeth.

Our bodies lose water every day when we breathe, perspire, urinate, and have bowel movements. During the night our bodies detox and use water to do this. As we age, our sense of thirst lessens, and the kidneys aren't able to conserve body water as well. Over the age of fifty, you may start to feel tired rather than thirsty and may opt for a nap instead of a tall glass of water. If you remain dehydrated, you can end up suffering complications.

A study was done in 2001 that dealt with the subject of influence of age, thirst, and fluid intake. It was discovered that even though older adults (over sixty-five years old) consume sufficient volumes of fluids on a daily basis, things changed when these older adults exercised more than usual in a warm environment: their bodies needed fluid and became dehydrated. Instead of drinking more fluid as they needed to, these older adults experienced decreased thirst sensation and reduced fluid intake. The study found that when the body is taxed by exercise in a warm environment, the full restoration of fluid balance is slowed. Thus, the study concluded that the aging process impairs physiological control systems which are associated with thirst and satiety.

SUPER AGER SUPPLEMENTS

To supplement or not to supplement, what choice would a Super Ager make? The types and range of supplements are vast and broad. In broad terms, pills, capsules, and soft gels are more difficult for the body to digest than powders diluted in liquids and or pastes. Also, there are vitamins and substances that are extracted of created in a lab. There are also many natural substances that are toxic or not so healthy, so please take care in what supplements you put into your body. As you age, digestion slows, so taking a paste, juice, or tea infused with herbs or vitamins may be a great way to ingest extra nutrients as you grow older.

Traditional cultures did not take vitamin pills, but instead relied on local herbs and superfoods. This would be a Super Ager's most practical and usually economical way to rejuvenate. There are so many choices and as a Yoga Health Coach, I like to defer to healthy habits as a first line of defense, especially if someone is not in optimal health. I will recommend that my client start with healthy habits, slowly building their habits for optimum sleep, digestion, exercise, and spiritual practice. If a person has all their healthy habits in place and they want to supplement for longevity, then I have no problem with it. I just often see clients, students, and friends who don't take great care of themselves and then try to stuff themselves with supplements. It's like building a house and that the foundation is healthy habits; if you don't have that foundation in place and you just start popping pills, it's like having a house that's tilted and then filling it with all these little tchotchkes. They might be cute and nice, but they're not really building your life. Once you get your foundation strong then you'll know exactly what to put in your house: you'll know exactly what to put in your body. You will feel intuitively what's right, but see the right practitioners now if you're in an emergency. If you're in a crisis mode, you should see a practitioner and they can help you work on the foundation as well as the supplements. Right here in this book for Super Agers we're talking about basic habits: once you've got the basic habits in place, supplement all you want. Habits are going to start to build the momentum and change your life you may need to do other things if you're in a crisis.

The "Clean Fifteen" and the "Dirty Dozen"

The Environmental Working Group (ewg.org) compiles two annual lists that can be helpful when selecting produce and eating out, the "Dirty Dozen" and the "Clean Fifteen."

- **Dirty Dozen** – Avoid these pesticide-ridden nonorganic fruits and vegetables as much as possible. Remember most restaurants do not use organic produce unless specified. These are: strawberries, spinach, nectarines, apples, peaches, pears, cherries, grapes, celery, tomatoes, sweet bell peppers, and potatoes.

- **Clean Fifteen** – These are the best nonorganic fruits and vegetables that you can buy because they contain the least amount of pesticides: sweet corn, avocados, pineapples, cabbage, onions, sweet peas (frozen), papayas, asparagus, mangos, eggplant, honeydew melon, kiwi, cantaloupe, cauliflower, and grapefruit.

Soil Makes a Difference, Where Your Food Grows

Minerals are inorganic substances that occur naturally in water, soil, rocks, plants, and animals. Plants grown in mineral rich, "healthy" soil will be more nutritious than those that are grown in depleted soil. Soil makes a difference, ask any wine producer about the effect that soil has on the final product of wine. Become a produce connoisseur. Just like someone who seeks out fine wines you can be someone who seeks out the healthiest produce. It will taste so much more delicious. Get to know those who produce your food and ask them about their farming practices. Most small and some larger organic farms tend their soil carefully. Go to Farmer's markets, grow your own fruits and vegetables buy from a CSA, or an urban farm and you will probably be find food grown in healthy well mineralized soil. Depleted soil will yield produce that is not nutrient-dense, especially in terms of minerals. Commercial farms typically produce vegetables and fruits that are not as high in vitamins and minerals. Try to buy from Biodynamic and organic farms.

Minerals build teeth, bones, blood, skin, and hair and help with nerve function. Minerals such as calcium and magnesium help to build bones and support muscle function. Trace minerals such as selenium and copper are required by the body in very small amounts.

Electrolytes are minerals that dissolve in water to form ions that help carry electrical impulses between cells. Potassium, sodium, chloride, calcium, and magnesium are ionic minerals that need to be balanced in the body. The electrolyte fluid balance in your cells is important, and if it is off-balance in your muscles you will get muscle cramps. Our cells use certain minerals together with water to carry electrical impulses through the body.

Plant-Based Food & Drink

There are a lot of different plant-based foods and drinks that can help with your health. Here are just a few:

- **Bitter Melon** – A healing food in India, Japan, and the Philippines, bitter melon has a curious effect on blood sugar and an astringent flavor, Bitter melon looks like it's covered in warts.

- **Root Vegetables like sweet potato, purple yams, etc**. – Root vegetables grow in the earth and naturally contain the earth element. As people get older, the earth element decreases. For this reason, root vegetables help to increase the property of earth in the body. Super Agers stay grounded with root vegetables, such as sweet potatoes, carrots, yams, purple yams, and baby potatoes.

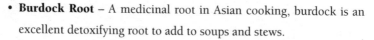

- **Burdock Root** – A medicinal root in Asian cooking, burdock is an excellent detoxifying root to add to soups and stews.

- **Radishes & Daikon** – These are very high in vitamin C.

- **Sprouts** – Sprouts are excellent age-slowing foods. Sprouts are seeds that have germinated, so they contain a burst of energy and are alkalizing and nutritious. When a seed or bean sprouts it is filled with a life-force energy that can be consumed. Sprouts to eat include pumpkin, fenugreek, pumpkin, mung, alfalfa, broccoli, lentil, adzuki beans, and many more. Broccoli sprouts have been found to contain thirty to fifty times the amount of phytonutrients in mature plants.

- **Vitamin E** – This is a powerful antioxidant can also be found in hazelnuts, Brazil nuts, peppers and Swiss chard, Sweet potatoes and olive oil. Almonds are one of the highest foods in vitamin E. Greens such as spinach, dandelion greens, and Swiss chard also contain vitamin E.

- **Sip warm water from a thermos throughout the day** – From the tradition of Ayurveda, we learn that we should sip warm water throughout the day as a daily detox. Water that is warm or hot does not need to be heated by the body and is believed to be a tool for detox. Of course, you can drink herbal tea or add lemon or lime to the warm water. The warm water habit can be an excellent immune booster during winter months.

- **Herbal Tea or Tisane** – There are so many excellent herbal teas to buy or brew yourself. Find your favorites and keep them on hand. They are made with flowers, bark, leaves, fruit, or spices.

- **Juices** – Fresh-squeezed or fresh-pressed vegetable or fruit juice are best, but all fruits and vegetables contain a high percentage of water and the water contained in fruits and vegetables have natural electrolytes, vitamins, phytonutrients, and other powerful healing substances. The best juice is juice you make at home or buy as freshly made juice. When juice sits on a shelf or is pasteurized, nutrient value and vitality are lost. Fresh-pressed juice with a long shelf life is definitely better than many other types of beverages, but homemade or freshly made is always best.

- **Tea** – Green tea, white tea, black tea, oolong tea, all teas caffeinated teas come from the *Camellias sinensis* plant, all other "teas" are herbal teas or tisanes. All caffeinated teas have antioxidant properties however, the caffeine will have a drying and diuretic effect on the body. According to Ayurveda, caffeinated teas will increase the air and ether qualities of life, so their effect will shift as we age. Just as we may not need to eat as much food, we may not tolerate caffeine in the same way as we age. Notice if caffeine is a habit or something that you can tolerate as you age.

- **Coffee** – Coffee is also high in antioxidants, yet high in caffeine. Again, Ayurveda cautions that caffeine will increase the qualities of air and ether, known as Vata, as we age. We want to take things slowly and calmly. If you can keep a steady quality in mind, body, and spirit while drinking coffee, then it may be OK for you. As you age, notice how coffee affects you. Are you drinking coffee or other caffeinated beverages to override deep fatigue, or is it a healing drink for you? Again, noticing and working with your individual constitution is critical.

SUPER AGER FOOD HABITS

Plan your meals, take fifteen minutes a week to plan a week of meals, whether it is for you or you and your family. Use pen and paper or choose an app.

Take one or more hours and prep veggies or make stews or beans that you can convert into fast and easy meals for the rest of the week. If you have more time, prepare a few meals in advance. Ayurveda traditionally recommends that food be prepared fresh daily; however, if food is homemade and made a few days in advance, that would be better than eating junk food because you didn't have time to make food. You can always garnish the food with fresh veggies and herbs.

–PLAN AHEAD–

Prep food or prepare all or as much of your meals daily at the same time every morning. The more we run our bodies and our lives like clockwork, the more we create space for fun, community, love, and other exciting activities. Many times, food is used to fill voids of loneliness or feelings of unfulfillment. The more you ground and solidify your daily routines, the more you can let go of any internal blocks that may create cravings for unnatural, unsupportive, less optimum foods. Use skillful and integrative habit-changing abilities that we have cultivated, and grow them gradually. If eating more plants for any reason feels very challenging, save these changes for later when you feel more positive or inspired.

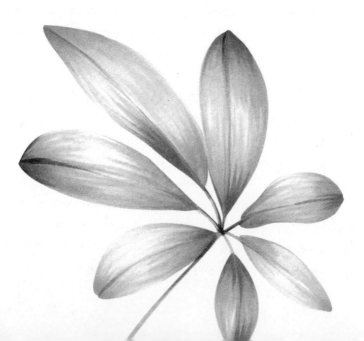

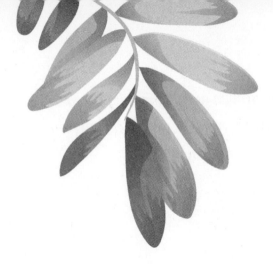

CHAPTER 7

**Surround Yourself with a
Circle of Support and a Few
Random Strangers**

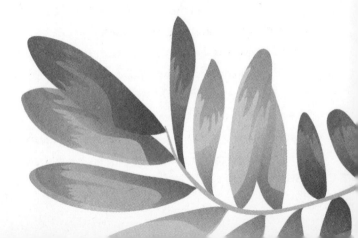

"The need for connection and community is primal, as fundamental for the need for air, water and food."

—Dean Ornish

In the modern world, social isolation is one of the biggest and least understood public health risks. And the peril of social isolation increases with age. Research has confirmed that the strength of our social connections profoundly affects our health. Lack of social relations has been shown to increase the odds of dying by 50 percent. Many people have a flawed game plan for aging when it comes to community. Often, they spend too much time thinking about the food they eat or getting enough exercise and fail to consider the effects of a supportive community. The good news is that your community can boost your health more than diet or exercise. And if you are someone who has some serious health issues and feel that your health is beyond your control, making friends, keeping friends, and building your community with new friends can be one of the most powerful ways to boost your health. The more people become educated on the health benefits of having close family and friends the more we can change the "epidemic" of isolation and the threat it poses to health.

In Ayurveda all that you think, do, and eat is interrelated. Love is equated with the element of earth. And as we age, we grow lighter and therefore need even more of this "earth" element. Your eternal nature, according to Ayurveda, thrives in a community atmosphere of love and connectivity. Aging represents the air element, requiring community and family help to balance the lightness of the elemental quality of aging. We need love to balance the lightness of air as we age. Family can provide a tremendous buffer against the stressors and the ups and downs of life. However, not all families are healthy. If you have a supportive and highly functional family, keep those strong ties. If family members don't support you in a way that feels comfortable, you may want to cultivate a strong and close a supportive group of friends or neighbors

A Librarian's Lifetime

Super-centenarian Bernie Nenner, age 110, has finally retired as a librarian. For several decades he stayed involved in his community by running a library at the Aston Gardens Senior Community in Parkland, Florida, where he is also a resident. Propagating a love of books and learning, he often quotes from one of his favorite books, *The Godfather*. His daily routine includes calisthenics and reading the news. For a long life, he recommends abstaining from red meat and smoking. "The rest is luck and the man upstairs," says Nenner. He has two children, a daughter age eighty-three and a son age eighty-eight. Nova Barret, a health care assistant who has worked with him for the past six years says of Nenner. "He is so kind. He's always helping someone." When asked what amazed him most in his lifetime, Nenner replied, "cell phones." Barret added, "Or as he likes to call it, the 'magic box.' "

THE MAGIC BOX

While the world now mainly depends on a "magic box" to communicate with friends and family, face-to-face contact boosts brain activity far more than Facetiming. And face-to-face contact actuates a string of health benefits. A study published in the *Journal of the American Geriatrics Society* examined 11,000 adults over the age of fifty for two years. Those that mainly communicated via phone calls, text messages, or email rather than meet with friends and family in person, had almost double the risk of depression. Paradoxically, those that sat down with friends and family at least three times a week were the least depressed. But don't toss out your device just yet. As a tool, when used carefully, a phone, tablet, or computer can help older adults connect, relate, and even help one meet up in person. Many adults have found support in grieving, understanding diagnoses, managing illnesses, healing, and supporting healthy habit change in online forums. Being able to connect with other likeminded people outside of the confines of time and space can be very helpful. Loved ones can Facetime with grandchildren, great-grandchildren and adult children. Someone diagnosed with a rare illness may find others who share the same diagnosis online. It's good not to throw the baby out with the bathwater, so to speak. The digital era offers some solutions for people who are isolated due to geography. Lean in to a digital community or forum if it helps you feel connected. Meet people in person for other social, health, and brain-boosting benefits.

One scientific study looked at Facebook users and longevity. Believe it or not, people who had a large number of friend requests and who also accepted all of those friend requests enjoyed a longer life. However, the study found that there was no connection to longevity for those who made numerous friend requests on Facebook. Could other people's friend requests demonstrate a likeability factor that increases longevity, or perhaps the act of receiving and accepting social advance boosts health? More research is needed on social media and its positive and negative effects on aging.

It's no coincidence that all five of the world's Blue Zones® areas are places that have strong traditional communities that revolve around interconnectedness, valuing both family and social family time. In all Blue Zones®, friends and family meetup in person at a minimum weekly and in many Blue Zones®, friends or family members meet daily or more than once a week. It's interesting to note that all, but one of the Blue Zones® are located in areas of the world that have been geographically cut off from the effects of modernization. Four of the world's Blue Zone® traditional cultures that value family, community and respect for elders survived because of geographic isolation. The only Blue Zone® in the United States is located in Loma Linda, California a hub for Seventh-day Adventists who are not geographically isolated. Instead the Adventists have intentionally created a sturdy framework for healthy aging through community. Every Sunday, all Seventh-day Adventists take the day off and enjoy time together. Although they do this in the context of a religious framework, their model of community offers hope for the health benefits of a strong intentionally created communities. The Seventh-day Adventist have a strong, values based culture. One value that would be wise to emulate is the Seventh-day Adventist custom of taking a sabbath or day of rest and worship. You may not be religious, but the health benefits of taking time off to relax and just be with friends and family cannot be matched by much else. Also, it takes commitment to stick to such a plan. You may feel overwhelmed and stressed and think you should work. But when you commit to taking a day off from work and career, you will notice the stress curbing effects of time off and you will guard that time in your calendar. Keep yourself unplugged if you can. Ask friends and family to do the same. If there is reluctance to disconnect, mention the Blue Zones®. All people in Blue Zones® spend many hours a week if not a day, unplugged and interacting in person.

Law of Protection of the Aged

It is not always possible to live near parents and grandparents, making visiting family a less frequent event. The tradition of Chinese Confucianism has a long history of honoring elders, yet even in China, filial piety has been eroding as children pursue careers that may take them far away from aging parents. It may seem odd to westerners, but the Chinese government stepped in and passed a law in 2013 requiring children to visit their parents and required employers to give their employees ample paid time off for such visits. The law cites the duties of children and their obligation to tend to "the spiritual needs of the elderly." Laws may or may not work to keep the family bonds strong, but education on the value of close ties may be what helps bring people together as we all age globally.

SOCIAL NETWORKING

As we age, our community serves many purposes. Some studies have demonstrated that our social network can predict our lifespan and healthspan even more than exercise. First social interactions have been shown to decrease stress at any age. Sense of belonging can often be tied to purpose. Many centenarians report their purpose as tied to some sort of social activity. In the book *Ikigai*, one centenarian from the village of longevity, Ogimi, Okinawa, describes her morning routine, "I say, 'Hello!' and 'See you later!' to the children on their way to school, and wave at everyone who goes by me in their car. 'Drive Safely!' I say. Between 7:20 a.m. and 8:15 a.m., I am outside on my feet the whole time, saying hello to people. Once everyone is gone, I go back inside. From Ogimi, Okinawa waves at everyone. Other centenarians from Ogimi describe their purpose as being with friends or "chatting or drinking tea with my neighbors."

Research bears out that our social ties will be a huge buffer and factor in the ability to live a longer, fulfilling life. Numerous studies have shown being active socially helps one to live longer. Support from family, friends, and neighbors decreases stress, and increases feelings of wellbeing. Developing social aptitude as we age and when we are young is an often overlooked marker of healthy aging. Healthy aging requires one to be able to ask for help and to be able to receive it. Social aptitude is not always recognized as a health booster, yet the ability to interact in an appropriate and healthy manner with family, friends, and even strangers does have remarkable benefits to our wellbeing. In modern western culture, society has prized individualism and advancement over cooperation. In Blue Zone® areas, older citizens have a different outlook. Teamwork is valued, collaboration is prized, and older adults are welcomed for their contribution to the community. People see the big picture of life and older adults are viewed as integral to the continuity of life.

In a scientific study published in the *Journal of Health and Social Behavior*, researchers discovered that older adults who had high or medium levels of social engagement and who increased social engagement over time developed cognitive and physical limitations linked with aging more slowly than those with lower levels of engagement. Another study revealed that socially isolated seniors end up visiting the doctor's office much more often than their socially active peers. Interacting with one's peers on a daily basis also helps to prevent a lot of mental health issues, which range from depression to poor cognitive function. Social activity engages your brain, maintains a sharp mind, and reduces potential for cognitive decline. Researchers also found that older adults who maintain regular social contact care more about their physical health. In conclusion, socially connected older adults have a smaller risk for Alzheimer's disease, cardiovascular disease, osteoporosis, rheumatoid arthritis, and even cancer than a senior who is socially isolated.

Social interaction acts as a brain and health booster; surprisingly, it is not just the support from close friends and families that keeps you healthy. It is good to interact with Lyft drivers, cashiers, classmates, and random strangers on the street. According to Dr. Claudia Kawas, lead researcher of the ninety+ study and professor of geriatric neurology at University of

California at Irvine, people don't realize or underestimate how much you use your brain to interact with people, especially those you don't know. When you meet a stranger on the street, you use your ability to visually process facial expressions to recognize if that individual is open, interested, trustworthy, and more. Then in speaking to a stranger, you must think of what to say, how to say it, when to say it, etc. It all sounds very obvious, yet if you are, say, fifty years older than that stranger, you may choose to say something different than a peer or someone twenty years younger. People don't realize how much mental work is involved in simple daily interactions. And many of us in big cities don't talk to our neighbors as much as people did in the past. The shock is how much these little interactions affect our health and life span. According to Kawas, "The more people outside of your own household you speak to any given month will lower your risk of death." The good news is that if you are mobile and in good health, you can improve your health simply by going out and talking to random strangers.

THE BLUE ZONES® PROJECTS

Blue Zones® Projects was launched in 2010 to leverage the power of community and local government to help people create and sustain healthy living habits. The Blue Zones® Projects works with communities to promote habits occur that naturally in Blue Zones® communities or areas of demographically documented longevity. Because environment often dictates healthy choices, change can come when a community pledges to create an environment and strategies that support healthy habits. The state of Iowa implemented the Blue Zones® Project in ten communities across the state. In these communities, local restaurants became "Blue Zone®" restaurants. Grocers displayed "Blue Zone®" foods rather than processed or sugary foods that might typically be a better sell. Local governments improved city streets to make areas more, "walkable." When a city, state or community adopts the Blue Zone® community programs, the program lasts about three years and focuses on local involvement through volunteering, structured community walks, or other forms of group exercise programs. The initiative's progress is measured by looking at markers such as reduced rates of obesity and smoking. Using the Blue Zone® "secrets," or nine characteristics that Dan Buettner found in the world's five Blue Zones®, the Blue Zone® Project strives to transform communities in the United States by affecting healthy choices. When surroundings and circumstances make it easy to make healthy choices, citizens increase longevity as well as quality of life, and the community gets an unintended boost as well.

The Blue Zones® Power 9® "secrets of longevity" include moving naturally, having a purpose, planting a slant, down shifting, belonging, and family first. The Blue Zone® Project asks the question, "Can Blue Zones® be blueprints for living longer and better in the US?" In an effort to leverage the power of community, Blue Zones® Projects work in conjunction with cities, states, and healthcare providers to develop community-themed projects in the US. "The people we surround ourselves with, even friends of friends, strongly influence our health." Blue Zone® Projects strive to create connections between individuals and community organizations to improve health outcomes for all. As part of a Blue Zones® Project in Albert Lea, Minnesota, people signed up to be a part of improvised groups in which members committed to volunteering as well as taking walks together. Even though other initiatives were launched in Albert Lea, the walking groups seems to have taken the strongest hold. In the five years following the initiation of the walking groups, surveys showed that the amount of walking done by participants increased by 70 percent. Smoking rates, are down and citizens of Albert Lea statistically have added an average of 2.9 years to their life. In addition, the town got an environmental upgrade, largely because the walking groups created a demand for safer streets and a more visually appealing cityscape in. Volunteerism drove mural projects in downtrodden areas as well as other cleanup projects. Research on telomeres, a known biomarker of aging, has shown that living in a clean, safe environment has been linked to longer telomeres and a possible increase in lifespan. Super Agers win again!

HEALTH AND RELATIONSHIPS

Most people want to experience a sustaining community around them as they age. Yet, discussing the merits of friendships and familial relationships is thought to be part of the realm of psychology and not a part of health care. Creating satisfying relationships that meet our human needs for love, affection, companionship, sex, and attention is crucial to healthy aging because the quality of our relationships greatly affects our physical health. Living in isolation as we age can be just as bad or worse than other health vices, such as smoking, heavy drinking, or eating junk food. The brain and body thrive when you age in an enriching and compassionate environment. In the book *The Neurogenesis Diet and Lifestyle*, by Brant Cortright, PhD, the author examines how our relationships affect our brain health in its chapter on the heart. Cortright goes into detail about research on relationships and reminds us that toxic relationships create more stress, while supportive and life-affirming, positive relationships help to boost neurogenesis, thereby increasing health and life expectancy.

In Ogimi, a village in Okinawa known as the longevity village, residents gather in small groups called *moai*. These moai support social cohesion and healthy aging, as well as purpose and joy in community. The Okinawan practice of forming moai was originally born out of survival. When times were tough and crops or finances grew lean, moais provided a community-based cushion and security. If one member of the moai suffered a financial setback or poor harvest, the group would pool resources and give the person in need money or food. Moai members pledged emotional, financial and social support to one another. Okinawans were traditionally farmers, so if one person in the moai had no food to harvest or had financial problems, the moai would give the member surplus produce or money that had been previously been collected. The gift of the moai seemed to have greatly exceeded its original purpose. Moais existence seems to have boosted longevity on the island. Although these groups were originally formed as a mechanism for collective survival, people now look to moais to have fun together and participate in recreational activities. Today a moai provides a sense of belonging and community support that seems to have a protective, longevity-boosting function for its members.

The moai model can provide inspiration for people in the west who want to examine our own ways of coming together and combating isolation as we age. We may have some communities or social groups that are supportive or fun, yet a moai is almost like a second family and has a degree of intimacy and interdependence that seems critical to healthy aging. In the book *Blue Zones®*, Dan Buettner visits with women who have been part of a moai for ninety-seven years. The average age of these women is 102. In Okinawa, people were grouped together in groups of five to help and support each other. The moai seem to have created a sort of community secret sauce longevity factor. Members of the moai feel more secure and connected, a critical factor in aging well. Those in these small groups report less stress and express a feeling of happiness and security. Small groups and communities help to depress stress and support the healthy aging habits of longevity. Another trait that may be supported by the moai is vulnerability. In the west and especially in the United States, individuality and personal power is valued over vulnerability. As people age, vulnerability increases, and without a supportive social structure to share these feelings and realities of aging, vulnerability can quickly become overwhelming, if you have never welcomed it as a human trait.

George Valiant, psychiatrist and director of *The Grant Study* that followed 268 Harvard students from 1939, concluded, "It's social aptitude, not intellectual brilliance or parental social class that leads to a well-adapted old age." The study was the longest-running study biosocial study of aging adults. Research from this study demonstrated that love in all forms has the power to help people bounce back as they age. The capacity to form warm and empathetic relationships could be the most important factor in longevity. Being connected to community means that we feel naturally integrated into a joyful, inspired social framework that includes both strong and weak bonds.

FINDING A COMMUNITY

What if yoga studios could become like community centers for those that want to embrace Super Aging? This could offer a solution to a few aging problems. I am a member of the Yogahealer community. We meet online and get together twice a year in person. I find incredible support in a group of likeminded people. Our group supports lifestyle habits from yoga and Ayurveda which can seem unusual in some communities. If your local social and family circles are not embracing the same healthy habits that you want to adopt, you may find support and understanding from an online community. It doesn't replace face-to-face contact, but support for specialized groups is something that many find helpful. For example, eating a bigger lunch and a small dinner is atypical in many western countries. In the Yogahealer and Yoga Health Coaching online groups, we frequently discuss solutions or ways to help each other to eat a large lunch and then have earlier, lighter dinner. Eating a big lunch is a behavior recommended in Ayurveda, yet if none of your family members, coworkers or friends eats a big lunch and a small dinner at 5 p.m., then you can feel pretty isolated. In our online group a person might ask, "What do you do when you have a work dinner that starts at 7:30 p.m.?" Others will offer their solutions online, such as "I eat before," or "I take the night off from my usual habit of having a light supper." It helps to have someone to bounce your ideas and healthy lifestyle habits off of, particularly if the habits you are choosing to change are not widely accepted. It also feels great to know that others have your back and may be in similar situations.

Other possible support groups could be lifestyle meetups, a weekly yoga studio potluck, Super Ager meetups, Ayurveda discussion groups, healthy living book clubs. These are just some ideas of groups to form or join to meet and socialize with likeminded healthy individuals. A supportive, grateful, and connected community provides the solid foundation for aging in place. Italian psychologist, Anna Scelzo interviewed twenty-nine nonagenarian and octogenarian residents of Cilento, Sardinia, and found that these elders were very close to their families. Often, they lived with relatives and had frequent visitors. Community begins with knowing how to have thriving relationships and how to form effective teams. In western culture, teamwork is not a skill that has been taught or passed down through generations. Those of us that were born in the twentieth century grew up in an era that esteemed individualism over the power of a group or family. Knowing how to trust, be vulnerable, and work with a group is something that we may need to develop as we age, especially if we grew up in a western culture.

THE BEST MEDICINE

Richard Overton, now the oldest living man in the United States and the oldest living veteran, lives in the same home that he built in 1947 after his return from serving in World War II. In his Veterans Day Speech in 2013, President Barack Obama said: "When the war ended, Richard headed home to Texas to a nation bitterly divided by race. And his service on the battlefield was not always matched by the respect that he deserved at home.

But this veteran held his head high. He carried on and lived his life with honor and dignity. He built his wife a house with his own two hands." Home Depot and Meals on Wheels came together to help him remodel his home so that he could "age in place" comfortably at age 111 years. He loves his neighborhood and as a local celebrity, he greets his community with great enthusiasm from his front porch. "I sit here and wave at them, and they wave at me," says Overton. Meals on Wheels began as a meal delivery service and has now branched out to helping older adults remodel homes for aging in place. Overton is a living testament to the power of social connection. His openhearted demeanor has trumped any of longevity drawbacks of his love of cigars and praline ice cream. His joy is infectious and seems to prove that love and gratitude are truly the best medicine.

AGING IN PLACE

Aging in place is a phrase that often used in the west to describe aging at home or moving to a place where the upheaval of moving as health declines is minimalized. Blue Zone® cultures "age in place" naturally, meaning that this is woven into the cultural fabric of aging. Everyone in the Blue Zone® cultures are interconnected, and so aging in place wouldn't be something that would not happen. In western, city-based cultures, aging in place is evaluated in terms of safeness of community, community life, spiritual centers or places of worship, community centers, schools, university or educational opportunities, museums, cultural events, concerts, theatrical venues, walkable areas, affordable transportation, emergency services, emergency or disaster preparedness, availability of health care, and support services. In cultures where older adults are living on into the 10th and 11th decade of life, these aging in place requirements are part of the community life of the culture in which these adults are already integrated members. Some older adults may live far away from children and grandchildren, and the older adults may not want to move to the location of extended family. They may feel comfortable living where they have always lived. Or perhaps children and grandchildren do not know or understand the value of older adults. They may not respect older adults, and so the older adult feels deeply uncomfortable relying on younger friends or family members who don't venerate the aging person. Let's take a look at some successful aging communities and see if we can tease out the qualities that belong to Super Agers so that we can successfully mimic and recreate what we need if we have not been lucky enough to be raised or to participate in a Super Ager culture. I believe it is possible and can be created. We can begin to cultivate a community that acts as a healthy garden for those who come after us. The garden may be neglected, but it is never too late to tend to the Super Ager community and the garden that represents this community.

Intergenerational relationships benefit all generations, young and old. In the Blue Zone® of the Greek island of Ikaria, elders are honored by all generations. Older adults have purpose and responsibility on the island, just like young people. On the island of Ikaria, there is a longstanding culture of community participation. During the Greek civil war, about 13,000 communists were exiled to the isolated island. Their communal spirit seemed to have quietly flourished here where other intentional communes faltered. Along with the laid back communal spirit, the island retains a sort of laissez-faire religiosity. Many on the island are Greek Orthodox and participate in many religious rituals, often loosely interpreted. The island's older adults help young children learn social skills, and young children help older adults to get in touch with their inner child. There is a kind of continuation and a deep connection that occurs when generations come together to learn and cooperate. In many Blue Zone® cultures, movement happens naturally and so do intergenerational relationships. As the population around the globe ages, there will be a potential for valued relationships for all generations. In a world that is changing quickly, connecting with those that have lived long provides rich instruction in how far we have come and where we might go. Remembering the past becomes even more critical as humanity surges forward at a breakneck speed.

A 2011, an AARP study found that 43 percent of all grandparents live more than two hundred miles from their grandchildren. Yet grandparents who live far from grandchildren, or older adults never had children, don't need to miss out on the value of intergenerational interaction. When families no longer facilitate all intergenerational interactions, community centers and nonprofits can step in and help organize reciprocal intergenerational relationships. Senior Corps is a government program that connects adults over 55 with various volunteering opportunities that help students of all ages succeed.

Globetrotting Grandmother

Virginia McLaurin, age 109, began volunteering as a Foster Grandparent with Senior Corps when she was in her early eighties. She continues to help students with reading and social skills, and mentors children with special needs at Roots Public Charter School in Washington, DC. On her 106th birthday, she made headlines when a video of her meeting with President Obama and First Lady Michelle Obama went viral. She danced and expressed her joy at coming to the White House in the city of her residence and meet President Obama and First Lady Michelle Obama. A few weeks later, she was honored for her over two and a half decades of volunteer work at Senior Corps. When she turned 107, 108, and 109 she enjoyed birthday parties with the Harlem Globetrotters who taught her to spin basketballs on her fingers and she was given her own Globetrotters jersey.

MAKING CONNECTIONS

Intergenerational daycare centers that mix seniors with preschool-aged kids show great promise to benefit all. ONEgeneration, a nonprofit in Encino, California, unites seniors, children, and young people in intergenerational programming, based on spontaneous and deliberate interactions between generations that unite and uplift all. High school students tutor older adults in computer skills such as Internet navigation and social media at ONEGeneration. Preschool-aged children and older adults come together and help one another build and enhance social skills at adult daycare and preschool programs. Older adults can model and teach the young children social skills such as respect for others and oneself. Seniors can benefit from the brain-boosting power of relating to a preschooler. As we age, our relational skills need upkeep and care, so interacting with preschoolers also has brain benefits for the older adults. The brain lights up in social interaction and face-to-face contact. Sometimes older adults get stuck in their ways, so interacting with young children can help stimulate the minds of older adults helping to spark brain growth. As more community centers and nonprofits are adopting an intergenerational model that benefits older adults and young children, the benefits will become more widely understood. One study compared three- and four-year-olds who participated in intergenerational daycare with 100 preschoolers in typical daycare and found that those that interacted with seniors were 11 months ahead of kids in standard daycare. In an era when many older adults live far from grandchildren or perhaps don't have grandchildren, the intergenerational daycare model helps to heal modern cultures that lack the strongly cohesive communities where intergenerational interactions are more deeply woven into the culture.

Many centenarians make it a point to interact with grandchildren and younger members of the community. Older adults can learn from young children who live for the present moment, and older adults can help young ones learn about life and help them nonjudgmentally learn manners and social norms.

Ask yourself a question: what kind of community do you want to be a part of as you age? Many centenarians see themselves as part of a bigger picture and enjoy the changes that they see around them. How can your life experience help society? How can you create a more holistic, equitable, and uplifting society? What would your Super Ager community look like? Would your community have many social or cultural events? Do you want to live in a city, a village, or in a more rural center? Do you want to live near nature, a park, a lake, or somewhere else? Do you want to attend concerts, educational, or arts events? It helps to tease out and prioritize your values and then reverse-engineer a way to connect in community with those who have similar interests and values.

I have spoken to some of my colleagues in Yoga Health Coaching and asked them how they envision getting older. What type of communities would they like to surround themselves with? Rachel, a mom in her early 40s, says she is looking into joining others to purchase property near her current residence in Arizona. As a highly functioning Super Ager, she is planning ahead, already envisioning her future. She told me she wants to have access to "wild areas." As a Yoga Health Coach and longtime yoga instructor, she understands the stages of life framed by Ayurveda. Rachel plans to be able to spend her Vata years in close proximity to nature and to be surrounded by family and likeminded people. What kind of life do you envision or are living right now? What is your community? Will you live in a city or the country? Who do you want around you? In many of the traditional Blue Zone® communities, family is extremely important. Yet in many places, people live many hundreds of miles from siblings, children, or parents. A strong family support system may not be possible, so an alternative plan is required. Still other may be estranged from our close relatives for a myriad of reasons. Many times, we may need to protect ourselves by creating boundaries from family members who may not be healthy for us. In this case, perhaps creating an alternative caring community would be helpful. Another Yoga Health Coach noticed that when she was in an airport, "everyone was holding a computer; all generations, everyone had a device." She wondered how this will change the world. Will people want more face-to-face time? How will our interactions change in the next thirty years? Will intergenerational community centers become common places? Will people become more or less digitally connected? What will community centers, senior centers, senior housing, and family living look like in the next thirty years? As Super Agers, many of us will be alive in 2050, and we must think of how we want to live in community in order to thrive.

-PRACTICE PLAN-

Daily Practices

Notice how many people you interact with on a daily basis. It is important to have both strong and weak ties. When you only interact with people you know very well, such as your immediate family, you often anticipate others' reactions. Our close relations often must endure our own prejudices. Implicit bias is most pronounced with immediate family members. This is where weak ties come in. You need to interact with people you don't know as well: weak ties. These are community members who you know, but not that well; you wave, say hi, and engage in small talk. Whenever you forge new ties or interact with these weak ties, this also boosts health and wellness. These relationships are less entrenched, so they can help you keep up with social skills.

Count the number of people you interact with on a daily basis face-to-face: can you increase this number, or do you need to? Can you invite people over, or do you need to go out more to meet with others? How can you increase your interaction with new people and people you don't know that well? Cultivate current relationships that nourish you. Seek out more people, both friends and family that you can rely on. And don't forget to meet with strangers too.

Weekly Practices

Engage in community activities such as volunteering for local causes or at events or arts venues.

Join a walking meet up or a class. Can you volunteer in your community or take a class? If you join a fitness class, you can get your body moving, your brain stimulated and create community all at the same time. Grab a play from Seventh-day Adventists: take one day off a week to simply unwind and be with family, or at least half a day. If you don't have family around, consider creating a small supportive group of friends that you can meet with once a week. Create your own coffee klatch, happy hour set, or modern day *moai*.

More Long-Term Habits and Skills to Build

Create a strong local alliance. As the world has "modernized" over the past few hundred years, in most areas close knit families that live in geographic proximity have eroded.

Develop a Sense of Humor

Make people want to be around you. Dan Buettner noticed that Okinawan centenarians were fun to be around. Everyone wanted to be near them and in their company. One teenager said she loved to be around her because she and she was funny.

Who Supports You?

How can you make intergenerational connections that are fun and help you and others? Where do you want to live, in a city, in the country, with friends, surrounded by family? Near a cultural center or a museum? Just as we need clarity about where we live, we will need clarity about what is important to us, and what our needs are, such as: skills to develop for healthy relationships, clarity in communication, boundaries, the ability to be vulnerable, humor, lack of need to blame or assign fault, letting go of being right, healthy self-esteem, not overly self-disparaging, and the ability to cultivate joy and inspiration. This list may seem obvious, yet as you grow old, social skills do require exercise. If you spend a lot of time alone, you will need to think of how to develop your social skills if they have deteriorated.

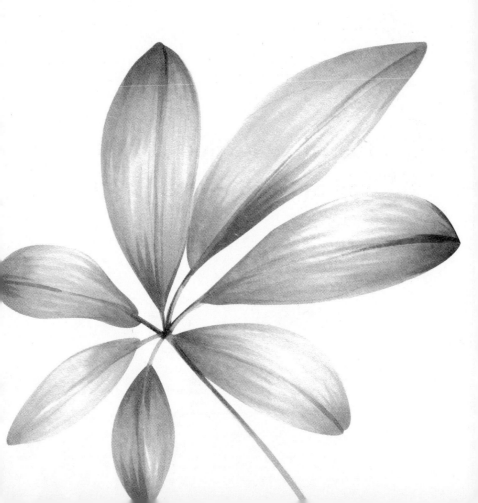

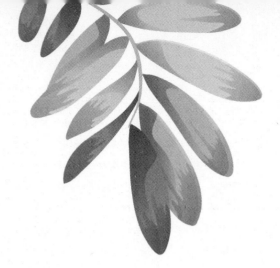

CHAPTER 8

The Ultimate Body, Mind, and Spirit Booster: Sleep

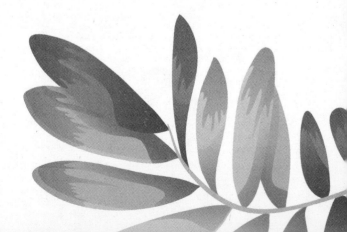

"Now I see the secret of making the best person: it is to grow in the open air and to eat and sleep with the earth."

—Walt Whitman

One of the deepest and most powerful ways to heal and rejuvenate your human physiology is to sleep. Yet sleep disorders generally increase with age, especially in the modern world. And many older adults give up on getting seven to nine hours of quality sleep per night because they feel frustrated. When sleep eludes you, do you give up? Do you throw up your hands and surrender to not having sleep? Or, instead, do you double down on sleep hygiene while attempting to get to the root of the problem? Knowing that sleep is critical to healthy aging and especially to optimal cognitive health is something we should remember and continually remind ourselves of. Dr. Dale Bredesen tells his ReCode patients, "We're going to treat you now like a competitive athlete." And competitive athletes know how much enough high quality sleep affects sports performance for the better. And the opposite is also true; when athletes don't get enough sleep, it causes a noticeable decline in their athletic ability. For this reason, professional athletes that encounter sleep problems are referred to a sleep specialist or health coach because of the critical nature of sleep. As you age, it might not be a bad idea to embrace Dr. Bredesen's approach to sleep health. Try to think about approaching sleep as if your career and daily performance depended on it. The truth is that advice is correct. And it is very possible to change your sleep habits and to sleep well, even later in life.

Super Agers aim for high quality, uninterrupted sleep. Sleep, the magic bullet for excellent health, costs nothing to those who "use it." It is one of the highest-performing Super Ager forms of medicine. No one will argue with the idea that optimal sleep will help you age well. The biggest question for most people is how you can optimize sleep and how you can get more of that sometimes elusive magic elixir of sound sleep.

As a Yoga Health Coach, my advice on sleep is rooted in Ayurveda and science. Ayurveda wisdom advises that one sleep adequately. In fact, Ayurveda dubs sleep one of the three pillars of health, alongside eating and love. During the Vata stage of life, you will need more sleep, and more high quality sleep. Read on for tips on getting the best sleep ever as you age.

Grandmother of the Glades

The legacy of Marjory Stoneman Douglas lives on because she took a stand for nature. Known as the Grandmother of the Glades, she was born in 1890. She first learned about the Florida Everglades as a reporter for the *Miami Herald*, when she was sent by her father, the founder of that newspaper, to report on the vast wet swamp-like land in the expanding area around Miami. One day her father assigned her to write a story on the first woman in Florida to enlist in WWI. When no one showed up to be interviewed, Marjory began chatting with the recruiter. Instead of calling in a story to her dad, she called to tell him that she was now the first woman in Florida to enlist. When she returned from her military service, she went back to her career as a journalist, where she was often called upon to report on the Everglades. As her interest and understanding of the delicate natural balance of the area grew, so did her advocacy of its protection. She didn't set out to defend nature and she often said she was not someone who was known to spend a great deal of time in nature. She was in the right place, at the right time, and became involved in making the Everglades a National Park.

In 1930, she traveled with prominent government officials and scientists to assess whether the Everglades should become a National Park. From a boat, the group watched the sunset and the moonrise and a spectacular sight of several thousand nesting birds descending on the Everglades. To be in nature and to watch the sunset and the moonrise is to be in sync with nature. Collectively, humans moved away from nature in the nineteenth and twentieth century, destroying and changing many natural areas. The drive for conservation and to create National Parks arose from a deep understanding that nature supports us. In 1947, Marjory Stoneman Douglas published the classic book, *The Everglades: River of Grass*. As a writer and researcher, she had come to understand the delicate balance of the ecosystem of the Everglades. As a fiction and nonfiction writer she developed a passion for causes that she came to understand in her work as a reporter. She championed women's rights, civil rights, and the preservation of the Florida Everglades. Marjory Stoneman Douglas lived to the age of 108, and her legacy as an activist for the delicate balance of nature in the form of the Everglades continues. She was a pioneer in conservation and raising consciousness. Her writing research and firsthand experience in nature led to her activism to preserve nature and the Everglades for over 100 years.

SLEEP AND HEALTH

Sleep is intimately tied to the circadian rhythms of the sun setting and the darkness of night. Living in balance and sync with nature is something that modern living makes easy to forget. Before digital devices, we lived in sync with nature. There was no disconnection to our circadian rhythm. The emerging field of circadian medicine emphasizes the importance of specific sleep- and mealtimes. As a pillar of health in Ayurveda, sleep acts as a substantial buffer to stress. For some people, a good night's sleep can be a keystone habit, meaning that when you don't get the amount of good sleep you need, other health habits may suffer. Many people feel physically, mentally, and emotionally off-balance when their sleep patterns suffer. Personally, I have struggled with sleep most of my adult life, but not until I strictly followed Ayurveda's sleep guidelines did I begin to get the long, uninterrupted sleep that my body so desperately craved. Ayurveda recommends some different ways to sleep, a little unusual for westerners, but perhaps not as much for traditional cultures.

What Is the Ayurvedic Clock?

The Ayurveda clock is a clock divided into six four-hour periods, each of which repeats twice over the course of a twenty-four-hour day. This double cycle goes from 10–2, 2–6, and 6–10; 10–2 is Pitta (fire), 2–6=Vata (air), and 6–10=Kapha (earth). Ayurveda recommends going to bed before 10p.m. In Ayurveda, when you go to bed early, and get up early you align with the rhythms of nature as well as your own natural circadian rhythms. If you have been staying up late and waking up late, you will find that when you change your schedule, you will often instantly become more productive and have more energy. You will get more done (at any age) and mentally feel very healthy. If you think of yourself as a night owl, it may seem impossible to switch to becoming an early bird. The truth is that changing your bedtime and waking time is surprisingly doable. To go to bed earlier, begin by changing your bedtime in very small increments, such as five, ten, or fifteen minutes earlier. If you gradually change your bedtime, it is much more likely to stick as a habit. Change it by five to fifteen minutes a week, or even every month. Soon you will be in bed much earlier and it is highly likely that you will be getting better sleep and feeling more tired when you go to sleep.

We just explained from an Ayurveda point of view why getting to bed early is so important: each day is a mirror of our lives. There is a microcosm in the macrocosm, and you can connect to it every day! Each day has a clock that aligns with your life. Starting at 6 a.m., the world goes into the earth period for four hours. This is a good time to get grounded, to exercise, have breakfast, and plan your day. If you are awake, you are productive and calm. The fire time of day ranges from 10 a.m.–2 p.m. At this time, the sun is highest in the sky and it's a good idea to eat your biggest meal. Then from 2–6 p.m. is the Air time of day. Creative tasks or communication might be great to try during this period. Meals, wake-up times, and bedtimes can be synced up with the beats of the daily rhythms. At night the cycle repeats itself. From 6 p.m.–10 p.m. is the Kapha stage. A good time to ground and process your day. Enjoy a meal with family: this is a time of bonding and connection. Kapha is love, glue, and earth. So, bond with friends and family, enjoy an evening meal, and then get to bed. 10 p.m.–2 a.m. is the Pitta or fire time of the night. When we sleep during this time, the element of fire helps to detoxify our organs and get everything in order. From 2–6 a.m. we return to the Vata or air stage of the night. When we wake up during this time, we can feel the expansion of the universe. The expression of the divine and we can get connected to something bigger as well as set up our day.

When you look at the Ayurveda clock, you can see that 6–10 is earth time. By going to bed before 10 p.m., you will fall asleep much more easily. The problem is that many of us do stimulating activities that keep us awake until after 10 and then the fire period begins, and it becomes very difficult to get to bed. Have you noticed or felt a second wind at 10 or 11 o'clock at night? For me, if I stay up past 10 p.m., my chances of falling asleep easily are greatly reduced. You will notice that you will become more active and restless when you stay up past ten. If you are reluctant to try going to bed earlier, I would simply advise that you try it sometime and just observe. But my experience with insomnia and as a night owl made me realize how hard it is to shift the ingrained habits of staying up late. If you compare eight hours of sleep that start after midnight and eight hours of sleep that begin at 10 p.m. or earlier, the quality of sleep that you will have experienced with hours before midnight is much higher than the later sleep that you have when you go to bed late and wake up late. The time between 2–6 a.m. is known as the Vata time, when dreams are strong because you are close to air and ether, the element that connects a person to universal consciousness. In fact, the time just before dawn is known as the *Brahmamuhurtha*. This is an auspicious time one and a half hours before dawn. Meditations and prayers are believed to be more potent at this time.

This clock can also line up with spiritual practice. The time before dawn is a time to align with the universe. It is a time for healing, because we can connect to the bigger picture. It is hard to conceive of the cycles of life and karma. The much bigger picture we can't really influence, but we can take charge of each cycle of the day and in this way take charge of our lives, our habits, and our karmas. There is a beautiful and poetic way to think of life and the dawn. One morning, I woke during the *Brahmamuhurtha* and saw a bright and magnificent shooting star—a beautiful reminder of the magic of the universe and the beauty of this early morning time. According to Ayurveda, the hours that you sleep before midnight count as double. Integrative neurologist Kulreet Chaudhary says, "Timing your sleep is like timing an investment in the stock market: it doesn't matter how much you invest, it matters when you invest." Health coach and author Shawn Stevenson refers to sleep time between 10 p.m.–2 a.m. as "money time." We can lose out on sleep cash, because now as humans we have the ability to override our body's circadian rhythms. Stevenson says, "Today, however, we can trump nature and light up our house like a Las Vegas stripper sign. We can be up until 2:00 a.m. doing the laptop lap-dance and not even think twice about it."

NIGHTTIME CLEANING

In 2013, researchers at the University of Rochester made a remarkable discovery, when they found that the brains of mice had a nighttime cleaning system. The brains of the mice shrank, while their glymphatic system removed toxic beta amyloids from the brain tissue like a nighttime janitorial service. Researchers discovered there was a difference in the way the cerebrospinal fluid moved through the brain when someone was conscious vs. unconscious. When you are in deep sleep, your body cleans the brain. Finally, a scientific explanation as to why we sleep! Lack of sleep has been linked with Alzheimer's, Parkinson's disease, and other long-term brain diseases. And lack of sleep can make you feel drugged and groggy. Lack of sleep has also been linked to depression, irritability, headaches, chronic fatigue, irritability, and weight gain. When researchers discovered the glymphatic cleaning system in 2013, that explained one of the reasons adequate sleep is linked to good health.

Many of the centenarians and older adults who live in Blue Zones® around the world wake up early and start their day with a morning routine that may include tea, prayers, chores, and breakfast. Routines can be individually crafted, yet going to bed early and arising early seems to be a common habit of healthy older adults around the world. A woman in Ogimi sang this song:

"To keep healthy and have a long life eat just a little of everything with relish, go to bed early, get up early, then go for a walk. We live each day with serenity and we enjoy the journey. To keep healthy and have a long life we get on well with all our friends. Spring, summer, fall, winter, we happily enjoy all the seasons. The secret is not to get distracted by how old the fingers are; from the fingers to the head and back once again. If you keep moving your fingers, working 100 years will come to you."

Get up early; watch the sunrise if you can. In every one of the Blue Zone® cultures, where the extraordinary elderly live, the centenarians typically get up at dawn. Many CEOs swear by rising before the sun, and an assortment of spiritual traditions call for followers to wake at dawn or earlier. When we get up early we synch up with Mother Nature—with the sun, the moon, and the cosmos. Getting up early can do no harm, unless you don't go to bed early. Getting up early costs nothing and it's worth a try.

RHYTHMIC LIVING

In Ayurveda, each season and each day has a quality and a rhythm. It's like being in tune or playing to the beat of a song. When your beat is off, the quality of your life is out of sync. Take a suggestion from traditional cultures and turn back the hands of time or the reverse the flow of the digital era. We can only guess what it was like to live as hunter-gatherers—or can we? A 2015 sleep study published in the *Journal of Current Biology* investigated the sleep schedules of some of the world's last remaining hunter-gatherer groups. Researchers discovered that all these tribes had surprisingly similar schedules. Although separated by thousands of miles, the San of Namibia, the Tsimane of Bolivia and the Hadza of Tanzania all woke at dawn and went to bed a few hours after sunset. Researchers believe this pattern was not an accident. This investigation was led by Dr. Jerome Siegal, sleep researcher and professor of psychiatry at University of California at Los Angeles. According to Siegal, "Seeing the same pattern in three groups separated by thousands of miles on two continents makes it pretty clear that this is the natural pattern." Because we can't go back in time to study sleep patterns before electrical light or digital devices, the study has particular significance. Dr. Siegal theorizes, "Many of us may be suffering from a disruption of this ancient pattern."

You will find your life transform radically just by going to bed early and waking up early. You are simply syncing up your body with the pulse of the planet, something that humans have done innately for thousands of years. Hal Elrod wrote *The Miracle Morning* based on the idea of getting up early, or at least earlier, to set the tone of your day. Elrod has a six-part plan to seize the day and get ready for miracles: SAVERS (Silence, Affirmations, Visualizations, Exercise, Reading, and Silence). When you take the time to focus on growth, especially in the morning, it sets the tone for the day, the month, the year, and the lifetime. It is truly miraculous. Filipe Castro advises the audience in his *TEDx* talk, "How Waking Up Every Day at 4.30 a.m. Can Change Your Life": "Try to push your limits well beyond your comfort zone, try to not stay comfortable, and with that reach things you never imagined before." He believes a small thing can start something much bigger. As a young entrepreneur, he started the hashtag #21earlydays. Starting your days early can be life-changing and at the same time quite challenging. As Filipe demonstrates, the earlier in life you start this habit, the better. And support helps, even from people you have never met: herein lies the power of the hashtag. Hashtags may seem silly, but when you want to wake up at 4:30 a.m. (or even 5 or 6 a.m., if you usually wake up hours later), looking or inspiration by seeking out others can be game-changing. Check out Filipe Castro's TEDx talk or look for #21earlydays to find others trying to get out of bed to seize the day.

Finally, the microcosm relates to the macrocosm. If you have been struggling with physical or mental health challenges for a long, long time, the morning may be your best ally. The microcosm of each day offers an opportunity to change our lives. In Ayurveda the microcosm of a day is the macrocosm of your life. Just as each time of life has an element, each day contains the same patterns. If you suffered early trauma or difficulties, the time you take in the morning to meditate, exercise, recite affirmations, and repattern your psyche will be most powerful. The miracle of getting up early is based on repatterning to reshape your day as well as your life. The time when you are sleeping signifies the time "in between," before you are born and after you die. The time of the morning is birth and early years. When we get up before dawn, we have the power to connect to that potency of this time. If you have experienced misfortunes in early childhood, or prenatal trauma, getting up early is one of the best ways to heal and transform early wounding. When you awaken in the morning before dawn to take time for your own growth-oriented spiritual or uplifting practices you can change deeply rooted patterns, even those that we may have acquired as a baby or even in the womb. This is the time when your brain is most plastic, and events have greater influence and weight. If this sounds farfetched to you, I urge you to try. It costs nothing to wake up early, and there are many ways to do it. Give it twenty-one days or more. Don't take my word for it: find a buddy or group of friends to begin waking up early. It's free, and it won't harm you if you get to bed early. Then let me know if it transforms you. In these pages, you will find many ideas on how to spend your morning hours, what to do that will work for you and your life.

Sleep and Light

Researchers believe that morning light plays a critical role in regulating sleep patterns, yet they aren't sure exactly how. Detectors in the eye sense light and then send a message to the suprachiasmatic nucleus or SCN, a tiny region in the brain located in the hypothalamus. The role of the SCN is to oversee the body's circadian rhythms. Light is detected by the SCN, in turn allowing for entrainment of one's biological rhythm to a twenty-four-hour cycle. Not all effects of morning light and entrainment are fully understood. Melatonin levels drop during daylight hours and levels of the sleep-inducing hormone melatonin have been shown to be suppressed by light exposure from electronic and digital sources. Research suggests that exposure to morning light may affect your circadian rhythm, so try to spend a few minutes outside every morning without sunglasses or UV blocking eye glasses.

Bedtime Routine

A regular bedtime routine can make or break our sleep cycles. Because most of us don't live in traditional hunter-gatherer cultures, you may be plagued by distractions at night, strange lights, sounds, stimulating conversations, and evening activities. This makes establishing a bedtime routine critical to long-term sleep stasis, to signal to your body that it's time to rest. Medical professionals refer to this as sleep hygiene. Your body needs signals and a routine to begin to wind down at night and to activate the parasympathetic nervous system's response for deep sleep. Like all habits, sleep needs a trigger. And in order to master our sleep cycles and quality sleep it helps to know our best personal triggers for sleep.

Something that you think of as relaxing might be like fingernails on a chalkboard to another person, and that person might be your spouse or child. Keep in mind, it typically takes an hour for the nervous system to wind down. If you conk out the minute you hit the pillow, you may actually be sleep deprived. A bedtime routine will help regulate your need for sleep; if you can't get through a thirty to sixty-minute routine without falling asleep, try going to bed earlier. Set an alarm or other trigger that indicates it is time to begin your bedtime routine. If you are trying to establish an earlier bedtime, try moving your bedtime up fifteen minutes a week, five minutes a day. Do the shift gradually so that you hardly notice. Plan for baby steps if you want to transform from night owl to early bird. Give yourself a year or more for a big change like this. Note that you are also changing a deeply embedded part of your identity, and this will cause some repercussions. Friends, family members, and even coworkers may express shock; you may feel you have lost a part of yourself. Usually you will be rewarded with deeper sleep, more vitality, and a sense of alignment with your own true nature. But even that will cause a stir, as the current culture does not always value such alignment.

Once you have set your nighttime alarm, it's time to begin your bedtime routine. There are so many fun sleep-inducing activities and rituals. You may want to choose a bath or foot bath, or perhaps a self-massage with Ayurvedic oil. Some people like to use calming essential oils such as lavender, sandalwood, and Roman chamomile. During your wind-down hour, you will want to reduce blue light that disrupts sleep patterns by delaying the release of the body's sleep hormone melatonin. Turn off all digital devices or use an app to reduce blue light. There are a number of ways to achieve the blocking of blue light. There are several apps that can be used to reduce blue light on digital devices, cell phones, and computers. One well-known app is called F(lux) and can be downloaded for free to any device. If you are having a family movie night and you have found yourself particularly sensitive to light emitted from screens, try purchasing a pair of blue-blocking sunglasses or amber glasses. Some people feel so sensitive to blue light that they need to wear amber glasses as soon as it gets dark. Everyone will be a little different, but don't be surprised if you become more sensitive as you switch to becoming someone who goes to bed early. If you find yourself particularly sensitive to blue light, wear your amber glasses one to two hours before bedtime, even if you are not looking at a screen. I sometimes find this helpful when hanging around others with less-stringent bedtime routines. If you look over at a TV or computer screen, it won't affect you. Another, more radical approach could be to do all activities by candlelight, at least an hour before bedtime. I have found this practice to be extremely relaxing and helpful during stressful periods of my life. Candlelight seems to induce sleepiness for many who have difficulty winding down. Other bedtime routines can include taking a hot bath or shower, or doing an oil massage (*abhyanga*). An abbreviated version of a full-body bath, could be a foot bath followed by a foot massage with essential oils. Often, people become numb to the stimulating activities, lights, and sounds that bombard them until they are gradually eliminated. Getting sound sleep as a reward will be worth it, I promise. And all of the same fun and stimulating activities can be moved to a different time of day—they don't have to be eliminated altogether. Sleep in a quiet, darkened room. Avoid drinking too many liquids before bed, because getting up in the middle of the night to go to the bathroom disrupts sleep. If there are noises that you cannot control, try using a white noise machine, a fan, and/or earplugs to block out sounds that may wake you during the night.

Morning Routine

A little-known secret-good sleep begins in the morning! Upon arising, go outside or look out the window if it is light. This will stop the production of melatonin in your suprachiasmatic nucleus. If you wake up before dawn during the *Brahmamuhurta* (an auspicious time an hour or so before dawn), meditate or practice yoga. Go outside as the sun rises or look out the window. Sleep researchers know that light affects our biological clocks and so influence our sleep cycles. If you are not currently waking up early, get out when you can and get some natural light on your eyes. Don't wear eyeglasses for the first ten minutes of your light exposure.

Exercise in the morning. Even if you like to exercise later in the day, try to do some type of invigorating morning exercise. Morning exercise has so many benefits, such as increased circulation to body and brain. As a part of your daily routine, some exercise done daily will be better than an erratic exercise routine, especially one done later in the day. Many Blue Zone® nonagenarians and octogenarians in Ogimi get up early and garden. In the Nicoya Peninsula, Blue Zone® older adults often tend to their gardens or take care of animals. In Sardinia, older men who are shepherds walk many miles a day with their sheep in the early and mid-morning. Being in sync with nature is part of a daily routine that helps you sleep more soundly.

Exercise comes naturally when you spend time outdoors gardening, walking, or tending to animals. If you live in a city, you can create a connection to nature by walking in a park or tending to a backyard or rooftop garden. If you have a dog, you will have a built-in routine walking your dog or taking your pets outdoors.

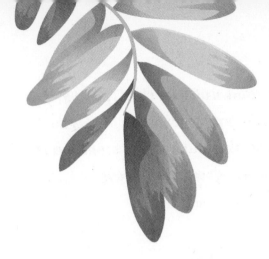

CHAPTER 9

The Importance of Creating Your Oasis of Calm Whenever and Wherever You Are

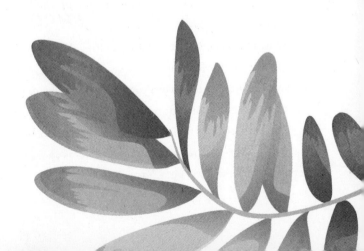

"If you want to relax, watch the clouds pass by, if you're lying on the grass, or sitting in front of the creek; just doing nothing and having those moments is what really rejuvenates the body."

—Miranda Kerr

Living a long, healthy, and balanced life requires relaxation. Developing the ability to wind down is a critical skill for healthy aging. If relaxation doesn't come naturally, you can develop the ability to de-stress at any age. And the more you relax, the better you become at the skill. When experts reverse-engineered the healthy lifestyle habits of the Blue Zones®, they came up with nine habits, known as the Power 9®. One of the nine healthy lifestyle habits of the Blue Zones® is to "Down Shift." In Ikaria, where people stay up late, they take a nap. In Okinawa, adults take a few moments each day to sit quietly and meditate and remember their ancestors. In Loma Linda, California, Seventh-day Adventists pray daily and spend all day Sunday enjoying leisure activities with family. Embrace unwinding as a skill. You can improve your ability to calm down gradually.

Many Blue Zone® cultures have practiced downshifting as an integral part of their lifestyle for hundreds of years. Having a go-to list of calming practices can help, because when you are feeling fearful or anxious, calming activities are not top of your mind. The anxious mind is predisposed to thinking more anxious thoughts, so breaking this habit loop will often be challenging. The good news is that this chapter is chock-full of relaxation techniques, practices, and ideas. You will want to take notes on which habits sound appealing and relaxing to you. These will be your go-to practices that stimulate your relaxation response and help you release destructive tension. As a restorative yoga teacher for over fifteen years, I delight in taking yoga students on a journey of letting go. One of my favorite pastimes is to look at someone's face and demeanor before practicing this soothing type of "do-nothing yoga" and then observe their calm faces as they walk out the door. When my students leave the room, they look literally years younger: furrowed brows melt away, and tense jaws turn into smiles. Anti-aging creams may do the trick on occasion, but my longevity tool kit relies heavily on the spa-like practices detailed here. If you grew up in the west or live a western type of life, relaxation may not have been integrated into your day-to-day existence. Try integrating soothing practices into day and evening routines, into monthly or weekly schedules. Take off your shoes, take a deep breath, and take a look in the mirror. You may notice a different feeling inside and out after doing these calming practices.

Prakriti

Prakriti can be translated as "original creation." You are an original creation. At the moment of creation, your prakriti is formed. You are the perfect mix, and that blend is your essential nature. In western medicine, medicine that is unique to a person is called precision medicine or individualized medicine. Ayurveda and many ancient modalities have emphasized a personalized approach to health care, which is now becoming a trend in western medicine. This is partly because of its efficacy, and partly because precision medicine can help keep costs down by eliminating the trial and error that many doctors have to employ to heal patients. And finally, the cost of lab tests has greatly diminished making it easy to use a battery of tests to personalize care. In Ayurveda, you can benefit by knowing your prakriti or "original creation." And what is helpful is that your prakriti is your mind-body constitution that never changes. You can use your constitution to determine how to eat, how to exercise, and even how to relax. Health is a return to your original expressive balance. Your prakriti is also sometimes known as your *dosha*.

Healing Songs

Mathi Mutu is 110 years old and lives in the Spice Mountains of India, just above Kerala. She always smiles. As a member of the Kani tribe, she proudly sings the traditional healing songs that have subjects such as respecting your environment and taking care of yourself. A few years ago, she was awarded by local officials for her work in preserving the musical heritage of her tribe. Besides sharing her musical gifts, she loves to adorn herself. Mathi wears intricate and colorful beaded necklaces, shiny bangle bracelets, and gold earrings. She is proud of her physical appearance and feels young at heart. She uses the medicinal power of touch and prayers to deities to heal many ailments of tribe members. Although many officials and family members affirm her age, there is no written record of her birth as she was not born in a hospital. Unfortunately, many demographers fail to recognize centenarians and super-centenarians such as Mathi. Written records were not a part of her heritage.

Traditional Healing

Professor Murali Nair is a professor of clinical social work at the University of Southern California Suzanne Dworak-Peck School of Social Work. He specializes in cross-cultural and cross-national field studies of centenarians and super-centenarians. He has interviewed individuals around the world who have lived over 100 to explore possible common longevity factors and practices. Nair also hopes that his work will bring legitimacy to traditional healing and health practices often met by disdain from western scientists. He says: "My dream is to bring traditional healers to our campus to sit down and listen to them." Originally from the state of Kerala in India, Nair grew up experiencing Ayurveda and other holistic traditions. While western medicine often scorns practices that hasn't been scientifically investigated, Indian scholars find American analysis equally funny. When Nair told Indian colleagues that scientific research is starting to show that spices like turmeric and cinnamon are good for your health, his colleagues laughed and said, "We've known for thousands of years that this works. It's a tradition that's passed along from generation to generation." After traveling to Canada, Hawaii, Bali, Hong Kong, India, Macau, and Peru to learn from centenarians, he discovered common traits. "They have a general air of optimism and positivity and try to instill that attitude in others around them," Nair said. "They engage in physical and mental activity on a daily basis, often cleaning, walking, gardening, cooking, reading, writing, and memorizing passages of poetry, stories, and life events. Learning never ends for them. They always hang around with people much younger than them. Even with a child, they find something to talk about."

SUPER AGER CALM PRACTICES

A primary practice in Ayurveda for healthy aging is *abhyanga*, meaning self-massage. Traditionally, Abhyanga is done with cold pressed oil, either before or after taking a shower. Using oil to massage your body can be straight forward, yet there are many techniques and tips that can help. There are many videos online, my favorite is a five-minute video by Banyan Botanicals (online at www.banyanbotanicals.com). Typically, you can do this practice daily, every other day, or weekly. Having a regular routine of lovingly taking care of your body by massaging it and creating connection and appreciation can be one of the most powerful self-healing tools available. Abhyanga does not cost much money and really doesn't take that much time. Doing abhyanga with a gentle, loving attitude can become one of the best life-/bio-hacks for aging. Aging can sometimes create a disconnect between mind and body. Your sense of touch is part of the Vata or air, the element that governs aging and this disconnect. When you massage and touch your skin with oil, you bring a heavy quality to your physical body that is needed to balance the aging process. You may have not been encouraged to create self-loving connection to your body. Self-massage for this reason is a simple and practical practice that will help you build a grounded relationship with your body at any age. Oil has a protective quality that helps you maintain energetic integrity. Your physical, mental, emotional, and subtle energy can become easily disturbed or agitated as you age. A simple daily practice of self-massage with oil can keep our mind, body, and emotions steady and focused.

Touch stimulates neurogenesis. Touch allows your nervous system to synchronize with another person. When you touch another person, you match energy: holding hands, relaxing, massaging, cuddling, or holding hands all help the brain. Touch releases oxytocin, especially during sex and orgasm. Oxytocin reduces cortisol, boosts immunity, reduces fatigue, and increases neurogenesis. Appropriate touch heals and helps the brain grow. When you trust and feel safe with the person that touches you or gives you a hug, you relax and further release oxytocin, inducing calm. As humans, we have evolved as social creatures. When we are touched in a loving way by another person, touch communicates safety. We feel protected and our nervous system relaxes.

Caring Cuddles

ICU Grandpa David Deutchman, age eighty-two, holds babies. He has been volunteering his baby-cradling services for the past twelve years in the Neonatal Intensive Care Unit at Children's Healthcare, Atlanta. Premature babies need to be held, cuddled, and caressed. The problem is that on-duty nurses and healthcare workers don't always have time to hold the preemies. And many parents have children at home, may be ill themselves, or have other circumstances that prevent them from spending time holding their newborn babies. This is where Deutchman steps in to serve: he loves holding the babies and says he gets so much out of his work at the hospital. However, society often attaches a stigma for men who are considered overly affectionate, for those that want to hold babies and give hugs. Perhaps he's touched a nerve in his unabashed love of babies. It seems people are tired of judging men for this kind of behavior. Last October, videos of him holding and singing to babies went viral and were aired on *The Today Show* and major news channels such as CNN. Deutchman says his friends remain mystified. "Some of my guy friends ask me what I do here, I tell them, 'I get puked on, I get peed on, it's great.' " They say why would you do that? They just don't get it, the kind of reward you get from holding a baby."

If you live alone, or don't have a spouse, lover, or family member to touch or hug you, there are other ways to receive touch, human contact, and love. One way would be to do *abhyanga* or self-massage; this can be especially powerful if you are in grief. Mourning a loved one can be quite difficult, especially a spouse or beloved. Loving self-massage may feel difficult at first. Eventually it will be a great tool of self-awareness and honor of your love for self and others.

Another possibility would be to get a massage. If you have an injury or physical pain, you may even qualify for medical massage that may be covered by insurance. Some massage schools offer discounted sessions with students who need to get experience working with clients. Sometimes even a fifteen-minute head or neck chair massage is a good place to start. If you haven't been touched in a while, it may take some practice to get back to trusting your body to receive touch. The need for affection is real, and sometimes as humans we shut down this desire.

Human-to-human contact triggers the release of oxytocin, known as the body's natural painkiller. While nothing can replace human contact, recent studies reveal that petting your dog also has positive health effects; lower blood pressure is the most significant. Experiments have shown that the blood pressure drops when you pet your dog versus talking to your dog. Not only is oxytocin released, but a number of other beneficial hormones are also released, such as beta-endorphins, prolactin, and dopamine. Best of all, these hormones were also elevated in dogs, making this a win-win for canines and humans! Mental conditions that contribute to high blood pressure, such as depression, could be reduced by simply spending some time with a dog. A few studies have also looked at the effects of dog owners' cognitive functions. Dog owners over age sixty-five performed better than non-dog owners on tests of cognitive function. Researchers believe the main reason for this was increased physical and mental activity which are related to walking the dog and the need to remember to walk and feed them.

If you don't have a dog but lack human or animal contact, consider volunteering at your local animal shelter. Rescued pets need affection as well as human contact, just like you.

Volunteering at your local animal shelter is a way to give and receive love to animals in need. The pets at the shelter need to be petted, and it will help both people and animals. A few years ago, I was taking my son to visit colleges in Southern California. On our visit to UC Riverside, during finals, we saw students lining up to go and pet dogs from the SPCA. A new form of stress relief during finals is for students to pet rescue dogs. "Take a Break, Pet a Dog" events during finals are popular for a reason. And animal therapy for older adults has exploded in the past few decades, with many organizations bringing dogs and other animals to help humans. Many hospitals and senior living centers bring in specially trained animals for residents and patients to pet and interact with. Adopting a dog or cat comes with responsibilities, if you are up for it. A pet can bring joy and unconditional love into your life. On the other hand, if you are not able to care for a pet, you can volunteer to pet and interact with animals waiting to be adopted. Dogs especially need attention from humans to remain healthy. Dogs that are waiting to be rescued need people to pet them. Otherwise, just like humans, dogs become less social and healthy when not receiving daily doses of affection.

Dry-Brushing (Garsana)

In Ayurveda, dry-brushing is known as *garsana*, and it has a number of positive effects. Dry-brushing improves skin quality by removing dead skin cells and stimulating the lymphatic system, which is also one of your body's most important pathways to detoxification. Because skin cells become stickier with age, older adults are able to get the most benefits from dry-brushing. Dry-brush daily or as little as once a week, preferably in the early in the morning, for its energizing effects.

Dry-brush by using raw silk gloves or a special long-handled soft (or medium-soft) dry-brush. It's highly recommended to do dry-brushing early in the morning, due to its energizing effects. Begin at your feet, massaging upward towards the heart. The same applies to arms. You are moving in the direction of the lymphatic system, towards the heart. Brush each part of the skin at least five times. On stomach, brush in a circular clockwise motion. The lymph vessels run just below the skin, and dry-brushing helps stimulate their normal flow within the body. By removing dead skin, the skin looks softer and younger looking.

Gently dry-brush the face to clean pores, remove dirt and oil, and reduce wrinkles. Dry-brushing the skin can also be a nice mindfulness exercise that can help improve the mind-body connection. Dry-brushing your skin can be a pleasant grounding exercise that improves your mind-body connection. Try it while practicing your breathing. The more you can be mindful and pay attention as you dry-brush, the better you will feel.

Essential Oils for Calm and Grounded Aging

Ylang Ylang Oil: Ylang Ylang oil is extracted from fresh flower petals of the ylang ylang tree, found mainly the rainforests of Indonesia, Philippines, Java, Sumatra, and Polynesia. Ylang ylang excels in supporting healthy skin, and research has demonstrated that it can help prevent signs of aging and skin irritation. Also, ylang ylang is a traditional depression fighter—it has a positive effect on the mood and it helps drive away anxiety and chronic stress. The oil also has an antiseptic effect that's great for clearing wounds and protecting them from bacteria and viruses. This floral essential oil also has positive health benefits for people suffering from high blood pressure. Ylang ylang oil can help to bring blood pressure back to normal levels. Use a few drops daily adding it to a carrier oil, or rub undiluted on your chest.

Sandalwood Essential Oil: Ayurveda declares that sandalwood brings excellence to whatever it touches. It's been shown to have positive effects on mental clarity and memory, and it has well-known anti-inflammatory and antiseptic properties. Its age-slowing effects come from its ability to prevent free radicals from causing damage in the body. For anti-aging benefits, it's best to apply sandalwood directly to the face using a carrier oil. As an essential oil, the aroma of sandalwood stimulates the sense of smell and the parasympathetic nervous system, meaning you relax and feel harmonious. Add it to your bath to let go of stress. There are several species of sandalwood that come from around the world. Indian sandalwood is best known and may be the most efficacious.

Take off Your Watch

In the words of yoga teacher Judith Lasater, "Take off your watch." When a yoga student in one of her classes or workshops wears a watch during yoga, she kindly requests the student to remove their watch. Watches can be a source of stress. The Blue Zone® island of Ikaria is isolated and difficult to get to. A culture developed on the island that allowed the residents to retain a way of life that does not depend on clocks, where people live life in stride with natural daily rhythms. Ikarians know how to relax. They don't use watches or clocks, but instead rely on the rhythm of the day. When we take more time daily to experience relaxation, stop rushing, and just be... we increase our body's ability to activate the parasympathetic nervous system, a.k.a. the "rest-and-digest response." It takes practice to activate the rest-and-digest response. Deep breathing with long exhalations as well as slow, enjoyable activities like restorative yoga are a few of the ways you can trigger the relaxation response, which helps to lower blood pressure, reduce anxiety, decrease our heart rate, and help us to *literally* "rest and digest." Herbert Benson coined the term "The Relaxation Response" in studies on Transcendental Meditation ("TM")in the 1960s. He wrote the book *The Relaxation Response* in 1975.

You may need your watch for many reasons, so try to set some special time aside each day or on weekends when you take off your watch. Take a practice tip from Ikarians and Seventh-day Adventists, who have no schedule on Sundays. During this time, allow yourself to set aside a schedule or to do list and let your mind, body, and spirit dictate your schedule. Do nothing but sit or lie around or do what pleases you in that moment. Remember, sometimes it takes time to learn or relearn to relax.

RESTORATIVE YOGA

Restorative Yoga is a form of restful renewal that uniquely rejuvenates the body, spirit, and nervous system. During restorative yoga, you arrange your body in positions that open and support the torso, head, and limbs in a restful way. In supported restorative yoga poses, the nervous system can enter the relaxation phase, creating for the possibility for restorative yoga practitioners to connect to potent vitality. One of my students aptly calls it "do-nothing" yoga. By reclining in supine postures and holding it in comfortable positions that support your bones, muscles and ligaments—using yoga bolsters, blocks and blankets to prop up your body—you can activate the parasympathetic nervous system to go from fight-or-flight mode to rest-and-digest mode. This essential transition is crucial for humans to master as they age. Because for the most part people in the west are often perpetually stuck in "fight-or-flight" mode (sympathetic nervous system activation). This activation of the sympathetic nervous system causes cellular damage, elevated cortisol, racing thoughts, and leads to countless other destructive behaviors.

"Rest and digest" mode (parasympathetic nervous system activation) allows you to metaphorically clear the mind and body of stress and thereby switch your body into repair mode. Note that the parasympathetic response is not the same as sleep. This is an important distinction, because you can sleep long hours and still have restless and unproductive sleep because your nervous systems remain stuck in sympathetic response, known as fight-or-flight mode.

What is Ama?

No, *ama* is not "Ask Me Anything" or "the American Music Awards." *Ama* is a word from Ayurveda that refers to toxins. The definition has broad meaning, and translated directly means undigested or uncooked. Ama can refer to mental or emotional stress, or it can refer to an actual poison such as mercury or lead. In Ayurveda, processing or letting go of stress is the same as detoxing from actual toxins. When you practice unwinding or relaxing, according to Ayurveda, you are letting go of ama. You may have old, "stored" trauma in your body. This would be considered ama and it can be released through healing work and Ayurvedic therapies. Ama is considered the cause of all disease by Ayurveda.

The ultimate goal of restorative yoga is for the person practicing restorative yoga to become deeply relaxed, yet to not fall asleep. And the most well-known restorative yoga pose is *savasana*. In restorative yoga, you practice variations of *savasana*, hence the name, "Do-Nothing Yoga." There are many classes across the country and all over the world: look for a certified, Relax and Renew® teacher at www.restorativeyogateachers.com.

Two Powerful Restorative Yoga Poses for Aging

Pose One for Super Aging – Rest and Digest

Take one relatively firm yoga blanket or other blanket, and fold it so it is about 24 inches across and 36 inches long. Make sure there is a defined edge on one of the sides of the blankets. Place the blanket on your yoga mat or on a carpeted floor. Put the blanket in a place on your mat or on the carpet to that you can have your head and shoulders on a soft surface as you lay over the blanket, with the bottom tips of your shoulder blades right below the hard, defined crease of the blanket. Bend your knees, and place your feet on the ground a little wider than hip distance apart. Ever so slightly, turn your toes in wider than your heels. If your knees don't naturally touch each other and rest on one another, move so that you can rest your knees together.

Soften your belly and breathe deeply. Spend at least fifteen minutes in this pose, preferably twenty to thirty minutes. It takes fifteen minutes for your body to switch from the sympathetic nervous system "fight-or-flight" response to the parasympathetic nervous system "rest-and-digest" response. For this reason, most yoga classes do not allow enough time for *savasana*. Try to go to restorative yoga classes where poses are held for at least twenty minutes, or practice these poses on your own.

Pose Two for Super Aging – Legs Up the Wall

Find a wall in your home or apartment that is unimpeded with artwork or other protrusions and take your legs up the wall. Grab a yoga mat or blanket, or do this in a carpeted room that softly supports your body. Lie on your back with your legs up the wall. Support your neck with a folded blanket and cover your eyes with an eye pillow or soft T-shirt. Note that if your hamstrings are tight, move further out from the wall and place a blanket or sweatshirt behind your heels to cushion your feet against the wall. There is a variation for back pain or very tight hamstrings: instead of taking your legs up the wall, use a chair. Grab a folding chair, or do the pose near a couch. Place the chair on your yoga mat or on the carpeted floor. Bend your knees and then move towards the chair or couch, resting your calves on the chair with your thighs perpendicular to the floor, or at a slight angle towards the chair. In this variation, your lower back is supported and there's less stretching or lengthening of the hamstrings which can sometimes aggravate the lower back. This gentler version of Legs Up the Wall will produce almost the same results as the first version.

MEMBERS-ONLY HEALTHCARE

Several startup healthcare companies offer a new model of health care. Join Parsley Health for $150 per month for a year, and you will receive a seventy-five-minute appointment with a Functional Medicine doctor, four follow up visits, advanced biomarker testing, five health coaching sessions and some valuable "perks." Pay an annual $150 membership and One Medical promises same day appointments. You won't wait long, in its chic and well-appointed waiting rooms, because no wait is part of why you join One Medical. In state of the art exam rooms, you will discuss your health with open minded physicians and Nurse Practitioners. Founded by an ex Google engineer, Forward has been called "health care with a dose of Apple, Netflix and AI" (Helft 2017). For a monthly fee, Forward offers medical tests, health coaching. More futuristic, than holistic, Forward's founder, Adrian Aoun was horrified by the state of health care when a relative was hospitalized for a heart condition. He saw doctors using post it notes and medical devices that looked like they were from the 1970s. As an engineer, Aoun commented, "The entire system looked to me like it had been frozen in time for decades. I was deeply disappointed by what I saw." Forward stresses data driven tools and 24/7 access. "We built a system to give our doctors superpowers. They use software that integrates all your data—from genetics, to blood testing, to sensors at home—to help you proactively instead of waiting for issues to arise," says founder Aoun. At most doctors' offices you will leave with prescription medication after 74 percent of your visits. Parsley Health boasts that only one in ten visits result in a prescription. Founded by Functional Medical physician Dr. Robin Berzin, Parsley Health stresses prevention. Why would you want to choose Parsley Health over a regular doctor? "Today 86 percent of disease is chronic and lifestyle driven." At a Functional Medicine practice like Parsley Health, you will learn how to take charge of your own health. Robin says: "My top tips for addressing stress in the moment are, number one, develop a breathing practice. … Develop something that is your 'go-to.' We know that if you inhale for, say, a count of three and you exhale for, say, a count of five, so that your exhale is longer than your inhale, we know that that activates your vagus nerve, which is your parasympathetic nervous system."

PRANAYAMA PRACTICES FOR SUPER AGERS

The breath is controlled by the ANS (Autonomic Nervous System), and your thoughts affect the ANS. If you are feeling anxious about something, your thoughts will trigger the ANS to speed up the heart rate, raise blood pressure, and increase the speed and shallowness of the breath. When this happens, you won't be able to think clearly. If this happens during a job interview, you won't be able to answer questions well. If it happens at a party, you will forget people's names or not be able to remember what you were going to say.

A Longer Exhale

The exhalation stimulates parasympathetic nervous system response. When you find yourself physically reacting to stressful thoughts, try some simple breathing techniques. During every inhalation the heart rate increases slightly and during the exhale, the heart rate decreases slightly. This happens for everyone in every breath. This differentiation between the inhale and the exhale happens as a result of the vagus nerve and chemical neurotransmitters that are stimulated by breathing. As a result, you can wake up the body by taking a shorter inhale or de-stress by taking a longer exhale. Take a breath in for a count of three. Each number can be followed by a word such as "one, Chicago, two, Chicago, three, Chicago," to slow the counts to one second. Inhale for a count of three and then exhale for a count of six. If that is too difficult, try inhaling for two and exhaling for four. Or if it is too easy, try inhaling for a count of four or more counts, and then double that count for your out breath to an exhale of eight. Easy does it—you don't want to strain your breath. If you are not breathing with ease, take a shorter inhale. Try the same breathing exercise as above, breathing out for longer than you breathe in. As you lengthen your exhalation, instead of breathing out normally, try to hum as you do it.

Deep breathing seems simple enough, yet try it. The unexperienced will often create effort in the breath and tend to breathe in the upper chest area. Here are a few tips I use to get my students to breathe diaphragmatically. Start by imagining you are drawing your breath lower in the body, like the belly or pelvis. You may want to imagine you are filling up your pelvis or even your legs as you breathe. Imagine from the waist down that your body is a type of balloon. Slowly and rhythmically fill the balloon that is the lower half of your body. When you reach capacity stop, do not force in any extra breath.

Full Diaphragmatic Breathing

Sit down and take three to five minutes to sit quietly noticing your breath and letting go of whatever is on your mind. For the breathing—take your hands on your lower ribs just above the waist. Imagine you are going to grab a big barrel in front of you with your hands. Notice how your thumb and fingers wrap around the invisible barrel. Next move your hands back to your waist. Keep your hands in the same position, but place your hands on your lower ribs, above your waist. Your thumbs should reach around towards your spine, and your other fingers can fan out around your lower ribs. Gently hold your ribs as low on the ribcage as you can, but still contacting your ribs. Now begin to breathe in and out, expanding the circumference of your lower ribs with each breath. You should feel your fingers expand maximally. If your fingers are not opening with each breath, work on increasing the expansion of your hands around your lower ribs. If your ribs are expanding below your hands, instead work on breathing as smoothly as possible. When you hold your ribs this way, you will feel your diaphragm expand, because it attaches to the lower ribs and incites deep breathing.

Nadi Shodhana

Alternate nostril breathing or *nadi shodhana* balances the left and right hemispheres of the brain and increases mental clarity. *Nadi* is a Sanskrit word that means, "channel" or "flow." *Shodhana* means purification. Nadi shodhana calms the nervous systems and balances the yin and yang of the body. How to practice: take a deep inhalation, followed by a gentle exhale. Continue taking a few more deep, conscious breaths, focusing on moving your breath down. When you breathe into your belly, you are not technically breathing into your belly. When your belly moves and expands as you breathe deeply, you are using your diaphragm, and that is a deep efficient breath. Once you have taken a few of these deep, efficient breaths, take the tip of your index and middle finger of your right hand and place them at the base of your thumb. This is *Vishnu mudra*. With your right hand in Vishnu mudra, place your right thumb on your right nostril and exhale through the left nostril, keeping the right nostril closed. Take a deep diaphragmatic breath (into the belly, metaphorically) through the left nostril. Now release the thumb from your nose and use your ring finger to close the left nostril. Exhale through the right nostril. Inhale deeply now through the left nostril. Continue switching nostrils repeatedly for about three to five minutes. Complete by exhaling through your left nostril. Take a few deep diaphragmatic breaths. Work up to doing nadi shodhana for up to ten to fifteen minutes.

Kapalabhati

In Sanskrit, *kapalabhati* means "shining skull." This breath improves circulation and sharpens the senses of smell, touch, taste, sight, and hearing. Kapalabhati improves cognitive function and boosts immunity. Don't do it if you have high or low blood pressure. Here's how to do it: Sit erect, with a long spine. Take a few full, deep, diaphragmatic breaths. Then take a deep breath in, and begin by quickly pulling the belly button in to exhale. Create quick, rhythmic contractions of the abdomen that last about one second. This practice is a little more advanced, so if something doesn't feel right or you don't quite get it, consult a yoga instructor. If you have never done kapalabhati you will want to start with a succession of twenty to thirty forceful exhalations, eventually building to about one hundred short exhale bursts. This pranayama builds abdominal strength. Remember to force only the exhalation.

Stress Response vs. Challenge Response

Shorter telomeres, a biomarker of aging, respond to stress. The good news is that stress resilience can be learned. When you reframe stress from a "threat" to a challenge, your biology shifts. Telomeres and the enzyme telomerase (the enzyme that elongates telomeres) stays with those who don't react with a "threat response" to stress. When you feel overwhelmed, blood vessels constrict, and levels of cortisol (the stress hormone) become elevated. One way to shift your mindset is through meditation and pranayama. Deep breathing and visualization can help reframe stress into challenge.

Telomeres don't stay long when you mind wanders or wish you were someone else. Telomeres seem to stay longer in people who are present and feel content. Cynical hostility can be one of the most telomere-shortening mental states. So, if you find yourself cynical or hostile (or both), consider working with a good yoga teacher, health coach, or therapist. One study showed that just saying or thinking about yourself in the third person helped to create distance without ignoring the negative emotion. For example: "Oh, Elise is feeling overwhelmed today." or "Joan is very angry at the moment." It is hard to avoid stress in the modern world. Understand that your response to stress can be trained through a variety of methods. Try cognitive behavioral therapy (CBT), especially for serious anxiety, dysfunctional emotions, and thoughts.

Chanting

A traditional practice in India, chanting has surprising benefits. Thirty-nine dementia caregivers whose average age was sixty did *Kirtan Kriya* (a chanting meditation) for twelve minutes a day for eight weeks. A control group listened to relaxing music for the same amount of time daily. Those that chanted were less depressed and showed improved cognitive function. Almost all indigenous cultures have chanting practices, including many African and Native American traditions. Aboriginal Australians used chanting to heal and Buddhist and Vedic chanting are widely practiced in many Asian as well as western countries. Chanting is believed to help purify the mind and elevate the spirit. Neuroscientist Marian Diamond found that chanting inhibited the release of stress hormones. Because chanting clears the mind, many report it leads to deeper sleep. Neuroscientist Dr. Alan Watkins showed that chanting helped to slow people's heart rates down and lowered subjects' blood pressure. If chanting it not your thing, try just listening to recorded chants to reduce stress and lower adrenaline levels. And finally, people caring for relatives with dementia were found to increase their telomerase by 43 percent after practicing a Kirtan Kriya or chanting and finger tapping for only twelve minutes a day for only two months.

Earthing

Take off your shoes and your socks. Next walk barefoot on the grass, in the sand or on the snow. You are now "Earthing." Connecting to the earth element has positive effects as you age. Why? One reason might come from Ayurveda, which hold that the air element that increases as you age is balanced by connection to the earth. In the case of "Earthing," you are literally connecting to the electrical conductivity of the surface of the planet. Proponents of barefoot standing and walking, known as "Earthing," include Dave Asprey, Dr. Joseph Mercola, and Tour de France cyclists. According to the *Journal of Environmental Public Health*, "Environmental medicine generally addresses environmental factors with a negative impact on human health. However, emerging scientific research has revealed a surprisingly positive and overlooked environmental factor on health: direct physical contact with the vast supply of electrons on the surface of the earth." Modern lifestyle separates humans from such contact. The research suggests that this disconnect may be a major contributor to physiological dysfunction and unwellness.

Reconnection with the earth's electrons has been found to promote intriguing physiological changes and subjective reports of wellbeing. Scientists believe you receive a charge of energy directly from the earth's electrons that helps your body to heal. Researchers believe that the earth's electrons act like antioxidants to help reduce inflammation and create other body-positive benefits. A review of the research on "Earthing" reveals a myriad of health perks, including improved glucose levels, elevated immune response, and reduced blood viscosity, as well as lowered pain and stress levels. "Earthing" even helped weight lifters recover faster. One study looked at Heart Rate Variability (HRV) by comparing real "Earthing" to fake "Earthing" sessions. People showed significant improvements in HRV after real "Earthing" sessions. It feels good and it costs nothing. More information on the theory and practice as well as products to ground your bed and other areas of your home can be found at www.earthing.com. Take off your shoes, go outdoors, and reap the benefits!

GET OUT INTO NATURE

One of the easiest, least expensive, and most beneficial practices for slowing aging and decreasing stress is to spend time in nature. In many of the world's Blue Zones®, people live in communion with the natural world, tending gardens, sheep, and eating produce grown on their own land. Most older adults in Blue Zone® cultures have spent a good chunk of their time connecting with nature during their life, and most of them have continued to abide in and lean into nature. For example, they are walking up hills or going to the ocean. Ayurveda's wisdom urges all people to create a powerful bond with nature. Many believe that God or the highest powers reside in the natural world. Spending time at the beach, in the mountains, or by a lake (inside of a forest) slows the mind and feeds the heart's furnace. Nature seems to envelop and observe with compassion our individual suffering, caress it, and release it to the wind, sweeping it away so we can be still and be held by the penultimate and ultimate Mother—Earth. If you have a dog, you may have a daily walking routine, which can oftentimes bring a canine companion animal into nature alongside you; it is not only beaches where there are more than one set of footsteps showing in the sand. There are angels among us, if we would but go and seek them quietly out in the outdoors... in the quiet places of our green and blue and orange-red world.

Forest Bathing

According to the EPA, the average American spends 87 percent of their life indoors and 6 percent more in a car. We don't spend much time outside. According to the *Journal of Environmental Psychology*, a 2013 study reported: "Short-term visits to urban nature areas have positive effects on stress relief." Because stress has a major impact on aging, forest bathing and spending time in nature may be something to invest in. This is another "free" therapy if you have the time. Taking time out in nature has also been linked to decreases in anxiety and rumination. Participants in a 2015 study who took a fifty-minute walk in nature around Stanford, California, scored higher in working memory performance and reported having less anxiety than a control group that walked for the same amount of time in an urban area. Forest bathers go to forested areas and simply bask in the light and air and atmosphere, sitting or standing in nature. Forest bathers report a myriad of positive effects. Connecting with the earth and nature has numerous mental, spiritual, and emotional health benefits that have been well known in traditional cultures. For aging adults, taking time in a forest can't hurt, and according to Ayurveda, the forest will increase the much-needed earth element. *Shinrin-yoku* is a Japanese word that means "taking in the forest atmosphere." In Japanese forest bathing, you take in the forest with all of your senses: sight, sound, smell, touch, and perhaps taste, if you find something edible. Studies in Japan found that stress hormones decreased after forest bathing. In addition, blood pressure and heart rates dropped after the practice. Ben Page, a certified forest therapy guide, runs a website called Shinrin-Yoku Los Angeles at www.shinrinyokula.com. You can reserve forest walks or find out more about the practice there.

SUPER AGER SKIN HABITS

Taking care of the skin on your face can have many benefits. Soft, glowing skin on your face can feel relaxing and boost a Super Ager's confidence. The skin derives both material and supple, subtle benefits from a healthy diet... and exercise. Another boost for your face is feeding the dermis (a.k.a. the top level of your skin) directly with topical food for the skin.

Super Ager Rejuvenating Facial Serum and Masks

Ingredients
- 30 drops of ylang ylang oil (we talked about that earlier)
- ¼ cup of borage oil
- ¼ cup of Evening Primrose oil

Directions
- Mix the ingredients in a small bowl or stainless-steel cup.
- Place this mixture into a small dropper bottle (an empty eyedrop bottle, perhaps) or into a squeeze bottle.
- Apply topically to the face nightly; being careful to avoid getting too close to eyes. Oil stings! If you get it in your eyes, consult medical advice or call a nurse or Google "eyewash," so you can save your poor

peepers from needless pain! And oil does aromatize, so perhaps use the cheekbones as the beach on which this mixture's waves will lap.

Manuka Honey Mask

Raw honey is packed with antioxidants, vitamins B and C, and live enzymes. Sephora stores sell a honey mask for $150, which ain't bad, but it's a bit pricey! Even with primo ingredients, the home alchemist can concocts an even better (and personalized!) one with your own ingredients for a fraction of the price.

Local Honey Mask

Ingredients

- 2 tablespoons Braggs Apple Cider Vinegar
- 2 tablespoons fresh lemon juice
- 1–3 teaspoons local or other raw honey
- Optional: ½ to 1 teaspoon ground ginger

Directions

- Mix ingredients in a small bowl whisking with a fork or whisk.
- Apply to your face for twenty minutes, rinse with warm water.

Manuka Honey Super Mask

Ingredients

- 1 and ½ tablespoons Manuka Honey[2]
- 2 tablespoons extra virgin coconut oil
- ½ to 1 teaspoons kelp powder or spirulina

---

2. The higher the dietary mg/kg of dietary methylglyoxal, the better. Manuka honey is definitely more expensive, but worth the price for its medicinal properties.

Directions

- Melt the coconut oil, place ingredients in a blender or whisk briskly with a fork until all ingredients are blended.
- Apply to your face and leave on for 20–30 minutes. Rinse with warm water.

Natural Brightening Mask

Ingredients

- One quarter to one half of a papaya
- 1 tablespoon fresh aloe gel (or processed aloe)

Directions

- Place ingredients in a blender, blend for 2 minutes.
- Apply to face. Leave on for 20 minutes, rinse with warm water.

Turmeric Face Mask

Ingredients

- 1 teaspoon fresh lemon juice
- ½ to 1 teaspoon powdered, organic turmeric (a wonder spice)
- ½ teaspoon Braggs Organic Apple Cider Vinegar (preferably organic, but apple cider vinegar is a cupboard standby that won't set you back too much)
- One quarter to one half of an avocado

Directions

- Put your ingredients into a bowl, and then mash with a fork until blended.
- Apply topically to the face for twenty minutes nightly or in the mornings, and then rinse your mask off with warm water.

SUPER AGER CALMING HABITS

You've read about many habits that can help you relax daily, weekly, and monthly. Aging well entails and embraces the ability to self soothe. Stress, loss, grief, and pain are inevitable. Life's ocean has waves; but how *you* handle life's little and big challenges has a tremendous effect on *how you age*. Start by taking stock of your habits:

What calming habits do you already have? What do you to relax? Do you need more time to relax? More inspiration? What would be your ideal day? That ideal day holds a clue to what would help you relax right now. Celebrate and remind yourself about all the wonderful self-care practices that you already do.

Next, consider the inventory of activities in this chapter that sounded inviting. What do you want to try? Make a calm practice time that you adhere to daily. And don't forget to do at least one practice every day!

What is one calming practice that you can begin to do daily? Don't worry, this can be something that takes only one to two minutes. This helps more than you think! Try adding calming practices to morning, midday or evening routines. Or perhaps you would prefer a longer weekend calm session. Spend one to five hours taking part in self-care rituals. Maybe Sunday afternoon in your backyard or every Wednesday night in your bathroom? Maybe it will be going to a restorative yoga class after work. If you feel indulgent, take a deep breath and remember that this is for you and your purpose. If you don't take care of yourself and take time to wind down, you will not contribute as effectively.

Practice poses from *Restore and Rebalance: Yoga for Deep Relaxation* by Judith Hanson Lasater.

Remember the Calgon commercial? "Take me away—Calgon!" Watch this commercial today, and you will laugh at the corny 1980s images of stress. But the mind and body can really benefit from that idea—taking a bath or doing something indulgent or relaxing can literally release relaxing yin hormones while diminishing the release of yang hormones which activate stress.

What action will make it so easy to do your daily spa habit? Maybe just having massage oil out in your bathroom will make it easy to give yourself a shoulder and neck massage. Keep your dry-brush gloves handy before you shower.

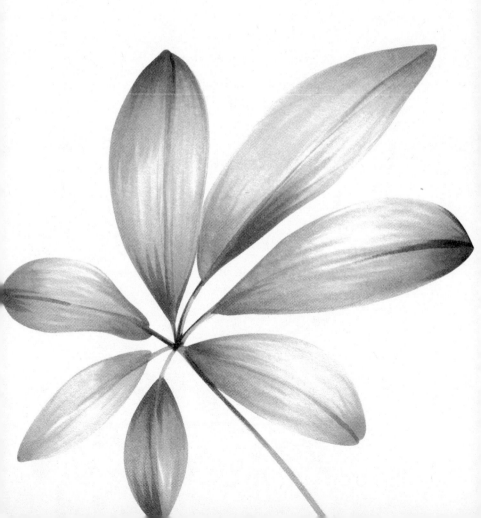

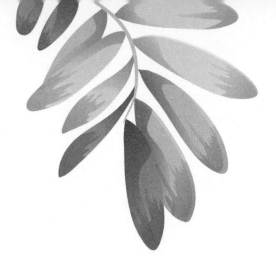

CHAPTER 10

Keep Your Brain Fit at Any Stage of Life

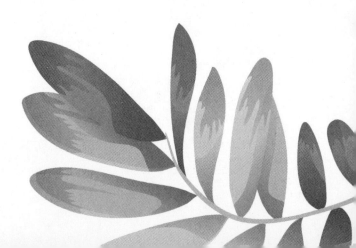

"You have the power within, at any age, to be better, more capable, continuously growing a progressively more interesting life."

—Dr. Michael Merzenich, Neuroscientist

How can we increase our mental capacity as we age? Let's start by understanding neurogenesis, the process of creating and integrating new neurons in the brain. Up until the late 1990s, scientists believed that the brain did not have the ability to grow new neurons and those that you did have got less flexible (or "plastic") after your early twenties. It was a widely accepted as fact that the number of brain cells that you were born with was all you had to work with. People thought that the brain you were born with was the only hand you were dealt. Yet nothing could be further from the truth. We now know that you can improve your "brain game" at any age. Research by Fred Gage, Marian Diamond, Michael Merzenich, and many others helped to create the foundation for an explosion of growth in how scientists understand the brain, how it grows, and how it remodels itself until the day we die. Because of these discoveries, we now know that brain health is very much within our control as we age.

Yet cognitive health does not occur in a vacuum. Exercise, food, a healthy environment, supportive community, and family all contribute to a healthy brain. In this chapter, you will learn about specific activities that will grow your brain cells. It should come as no surprise that what comes around goes around. When you activate the growth of new brain cells or neurons, your whole body benefits. When you grow your hippocampus, the center for memory and organization of the brain, all physiological systems benefit. Brain health is another chicken or the egg system of aging. When you keep your brain healthy, your body stays healthy and vice versa, with rare exception.

When it comes to brain exercises, as in almost any area of Super Aging, choose what works for you. If you like learning languages, sign up for a Spanish class. If you love music, learn to sing. If you enjoy sports, take up a new one, especially one that involves quick reaction time.

Rhyming Strong

Online trolls are typically a quarter the age of Larry Eisenberg, ninety-eight, a prolific comment writer for the *New York Times*. Technically not a troll, his comments are composed as limericks. An intrepid New Yorker, biomed engineer and award-winning science fiction writer, "He's the closest thing this paper has to a poet in residence." said of Andrew Rosenthal of the New York Times. Look for his witty, sharp verses peppered throughout the online version of the New York Times. I will leave you with his limerick posted in 2010, at the bottom of an article titled, *Living to 100:*

> As a nonagenarian, I,
> View centenarians with a sigh,
> Long odds, it appears,
> To live ten more years
> But I'm planning to give it a try.

Eight years later he's still rhyming strong. Does Larry Eisenberg realize the brain growing benefits of his daily poems?

According to Dr. Michael Merzenich, "most older brains are neglected." They become, "slower, less accurate and do a poorer job of recording useful information and controlling their owners actions." The good news is that your brain can grow. Just like a farmer, you will need to know how and what to grow in your brain. Neurogenesis or the formation of brain cells occurs in two places in the brain, the olfactory bulb and the hippocampus. Just as when you plant seeds, not all sprouts survive and not all freshly created neurons survive. The term neurogenesis more accurately describes both the process of the creation of new neurons and then the subsequent nurturing of these new neurons as they survive or die and finally become integrated into circuits in the brain. A farmer plants many seeds because not all will survive into healthy and mature plants. The brain also plants many seeds and naturally prunes back unused neurons and areas of the brain that it deems unimportant.

Brain aging and brain disorders occur when there are more neurons being pruned or reduced than new neurons are being created. If we think of the farm metaphor, sometimes there's a draught and we need to get more water to the garden. If we can't get water to the farm, plants or trees will die. No fertilizer or sunshine will also affect the rate of growth and survival of the new neurons. The brain needs a number of different things to thrive. If a brain has been damaged, much like a neglected farm, lots of attention care, nutrition, daily practices, exercise and stimulation is required to bring life back to the farm. Good things for the brain farm include meditation, a brain healthy diet, sleep, exercise, aerobic exercise, and mentally stimulating brain "exercises."

If you still have a hard time believing you can build new brain cells, it's good to know about the study of London cabbies who spend more than three years memorizing the spaghetti like maze of streets of this ancient and large city. An earlier study established that the London taxi drivers had larger a hippocampus than an average British person. Scientists weren't sure if the profession attracted people with excellent memories and large hippocampal volume, or if the job itself helped the brain to grow. It wasn't clear until another study followed a group of seventy-nine aspiring drivers for four years and found that that the navigational training of London cab drivers significantly increased the size of their hippocampus. London cab drivers made their neuron generating hippocampi noticeably larger after a four-year mental workout in which they were required to memorize the spatial relationship of an extraordinarily complex matrix of streets in London. Researchers concluded that "brain training" has the potential to literally enlarge your brain. It's the area of the brain responsible for organizing memory and neurogenesis. The taxi drivers were not just memorizing a vocab list, they were remembering visual and spatial information, associated with navigation. When you remember how streets are organized, or you can recall an overview of navigation to a location to a place from where you are at the moment (think GPS but in your mind.) Spatial memory has a different effect on the brain. Take time off from Waze or Google maps and navigate with electronic devices. It can be one best workouts for your brain.

"If you want to train your muscles to be strong, fast or to endure, then you have to have certain kinds of training. Most people didn't think of the brain in the same way until the past few decades. But now suddenly, with this plasticity model, we're saying no, hold it, we can design specific tailored therapies for individual to exercise their brain in a certain way to generate neurogenesis."
—Dr. Jeffrey Bland, *The Broken Brain*

As we age, fluid, process-based intelligence declines more quickly than crystallized abilities or abilities based on accumulated knowledge. Processing speed slows, unless we do activities or brain exercises that help to stop or slow the slowing down of our brain. Unfortunately, a typical scenario happens when older adults realize that it takes more time to perceive, interpret and execute responses to questions, or to react in certain situations, such as on the job, or in a relationship. As a result, the older adult begins to shy away from activities that are more challenging to their brains. And unless the older adult knows that all the slowing can be improved, many times a negative thought process arises. "Oh, I am getting old." or "I can't do math like I used to." Those who are employed may start to shirk away from tasks or activities that may demonstrate their cognitive decline. Maybe the older adult does not want younger colleagues to think that he/she is getting old or slow. Ironically as you age, you should do just the opposite of avoiding mental challenges. The minute you notice cognitive losses, you would do best to amp up your personal brain training and stimulate rather your brain, rather than decrease input out of fear.

Dr. Michael Merzenich tells a great story about his mother-in-law's pie making ability to illustrate this point. Baking a pie is a refined art. It can be challenging to get the crust flaky and just right. Perception and processing speed are critical to pie making and cooking for that matter. In fact, baking and cooking are great brain-boosting skills. Dr. Merzenich's mother-in-law began to notice a deterioration in her pie making skills, yet instead of grabbing her measuring cups and doubling down on her dessert making aptitude, she became ashamed. No longer would she triumph at the next bake off, she thought to herself. And so began her mental retreat from pastry making. She feared, her pies just weren't up to snuff. And guess what? Her fear became a self-fulfilling prophecy. Because her tarts weren't as good as they used to be she stopped practicing. She quit. By doing this she insured that she would never return to the pie making success of her younger brain days. This is the use it or lose of the aging brain. World class musicians face the same dilemma. If you are an amazingly skilled guitarist, you may notice a slight drop in your proficiency as you age. Yet at that point you have a profound and important choice, quit or practice a little bit harder. By adding more rehearsals, any musician can keep up their skills as they age. The same goes for all of us. You must remember it may take you a little more mental elbow grease to get through the challenge period. Resilience becomes a critical factor for brain health as you age. Super Agers just keep on learning.

BECOMING A CARICATURE OF YOURSELF

Social Skills as you age can deteriorate, just like cognitive function. In fact, it is cognitive function that is causing social skills to become degraded. As we age we lose the gray areas and often become over confident and lack the ability to ask for feedback. If we tend towards self-effacement, we may need to realize this and "Just Do It" or perhaps recite affirmations to our self. More confident older adults can become insensitive to their brash behavior. Both of these behaviors, becoming overly timid or becoming overly arrogant are a natural part of the brain's pruning system. If you are more timid, your brain will reinforce that. If you tend to be bold, the brain will reinforce that behavior. You will need to temper the nuances as you age. To do that get out of your comfort zone. If you are shy and not as confident, force yourself to speak up and assert yourself. And if you tend to be a bit obnoxious or think you have that tendency. Try your best to learn how to be humble. Ask for feedback from friends and relatives who know you well if you think you are missing the nuances of your personality. Get feedback. This can be awkward, so only ask friends and family members that you trust. Ask questions such as, "Do you think I could be more confident?" or "Do you think I am being overly confident?"

Keeping up with your craft, so to speak can be crucial to brain health. It is one of the reasons that older artists that take care of themselves and keep up their work have lifestyle buffers that many don't take advantage of. Whether you are a musician, a ceramic artist or you simply want to begin writing poetry, the brain-boosting power of the arts should encourage you to pursue the creative challenges that inspire your soul.

A Living Legend

Whang-od Oggay, age 101, is a tattoo artist, or *mambabatok*, from Buscalin, Kalinga, in the Philippines. She learned the sacred art when she was just fifteen years old. Originally the hand-tapped tattoos were only for *Butbut* warriors, and that employ thorns and natural dyes. More than eighty-five years later, she continues to create tattoos by tapping a dye covered thorn onto the skin to create a nature inspired design or geometric shape. Some designs represent the mountains, the sun, fertility and strength. Typically, this form of traditional skin art would be transferred through direct lineage, but because Whang-od has no children, she decided to train two of her grandnieces in the art. GPS won't work in Buscalin, Kalinga. Many Filipinos and foreigners make the journey by hiring a guide to bring them to Whang-od to get a tattoo from her or one of her apprentices. Her hands are steady and at 101 and she plans to continue her work, "As long as I can see well, I will keep giving tattoos. I'll stop once my vision gets blurry." Last year she traveled by helicopter via the Philippine Air Force to Manila to receive a living legend award, and meet her favorite Filipino actor, Coco Martin. She presented at a cultural festival with her grandnieces demonstrating traditional Kalinga tattoo techniques, using bamboo sticks, pomelo thorns, water and charcoal. Her secret to longevity: "I don't eat canned foods with oil or preservatives. I only eat organic foods, like leafy vegetable and beans."

Research has shown that by interacting with others, we actually train our brains. Social motivation and social contact can improve memory formation and recall. "Face-to-face contact is like a vaccine," Psychologist Susan Pinker, author of *The Village Effect*, affirms that direct person-to-person contact triggers parts of our brain that release a "cocktail" of neurotransmitters tasked with regulating our response to stress and anxiety and protects the brain from neurodegenerative diseases. And lifelong learners and teachers take note! When you learn something with the purpose of teaching or sharing your knowledge others, you learn more effectively. Prof. Matthew Lieberman of Neuroscience at University of California, Los Angeles specializes in the mechanics of what he calls our "social brain," the neural activity related to social interaction, and the brain benefits derived from them. His research indicates that "if you learn in order to teach someone else, then you learn better than if you learn in order to take a test." This goes against the prominent beliefs in modern educational systems, in which learning on one's own, for the sake of accumulating knowledge and skills, is typically preferred. Super Agers learn so they can teach.

BRAIN BOOT CAMP

Why do people in cognitively stimulating occupations exhibit greater skills in memory, intellectual flexibility, verbal abilities and fluency? It seems that the more you stimulate your mind, the better it functions as you age. Pilots, college professors, physicians, musicians and architects keep perform at a higher cognitive level than same age peers. Keeping your brain sharp takes work and intellectual stimulation comes in many forms. Older adults who play chess and bridge score higher on working memory and reasoning tests than nonplayers.

Below are many ideas for mental pushups and neuron crunches that will keep your brain healthy. Increase the speed that fires your synapses. Work out your gray matter so that you re-organize your neurocircuits. Do these brain exercises. Bonus benefits come when you teach others about your brain boot camp workouts.

- Exercise is known for increasing BDNF, the substances that has been dubbed by Dr. Mark Hyman as "Miracle Grow" for the Brain. Chapter 5 contains many forms of exercise that help your mind. Boost your brain by taking a daily of twenty minutes or more. And with walking, you can add on many brain "bonuses" that will enhance memory and grow your gray matter. Practice these boosts to your daily walk or add them on some days. 1. While you walk, pay attention to your senses. Turn off that podcast or Spotify playlist. Walk in nature if you can, and instead of zoning out or listening to music, press record on your brain. Here's why, remember a walk you took while you were on vacation. Often you remember every detail because the vacation hike was a novel situation and new things turn our brain plasticity switches on. When you do the same walk every day, your brain goes on autopilot. Fortunately, you have the power to cue the brain. You can tell your mind that this is a very special walk and they remember it. That's all you have to do is to tell yourself this is very important, as though your life depends on it. Imagine you are walking with a toddler, marvel in the details. Be mindful and pay attention. Pretend you are a toddler and everything you see and do is new and exciting. Wherever you are, listen to the sounds around you, notice the colors around you with your eyes, smell the scents. Feel the sun, the wind or other weather conditions on your skin. Notice how your body moves in space. When you engage your senses and pay attention, the brain comes to life like a Christmas tree. Running on a treadmill while you binge watch Netflix will increase neurogenesis, because aerobic exercise stimulates the growth of new neurons. But, you won't build any other area of the brain. The best and most efficient way to grow your neurons is to take a mindful walk and pay attention to as many of your senses as you can. If you brain does not think your walk was important, it literally doesn't get saved, the neurons go in the trash. Subsequently when we practice our skills in remembering what we did, we grow the brain and keep it healthy.

- When you arrive home after your walk or later in the day, do a mental recap of your walk. Use your mind to remember and jog your recall skills. Do one of more of the following exercises. Draw a detailed map of where your earlier walk took place. This could be done immediately following or at another time during the day. Draw either a map of the area, or one street, a tree, a sign or something that caught your attention. Add colors to your recall. Paint a picture of a beautiful tree, flower or other object you so along the way. Using your recollection abilities will activate and strengthen the brain's ability to reconstruct events and objects from memory. Visual recall and recording will be like deep squats for your gray matter. Finally, for those who want to increase cyclical rhythm, walk at sunrise or early in the day. The early light affects the brain's circadian clock and helps you to sleep better at night. Early walks have always been recommended for mental health in Ayurveda.

- Gamify brain training—think video games are just for kids? Believe it or not online computer brain training programs have been scientifically documented to improve cognitive function. Designed to help keep the brain on point, most online training systems are designed to meet you where you are. After an initial assessment of processing speed, and other cognitive values, you begin play. Surprisingly fun and challenging, the games change as your brain changes. Many people report better short-term memory and word recall after just a few weeks of online brain training. One study showed an astonishing decrease in Alzheimer's disease and improved cognitive function even 5 years after only a 10-week brain training program. Brain HQ by Posit Science offers brain training exercises, "clinically proven to improve cognitive performance." Online brain training sharpens reaction time, multiple object tracking, memory, visual acuity, processing speed and peripheral vision, all skills that can decline with age. Drivesharp, another science based, brain training system helps drivers hone driving skills that often decline with age. In one study of Drivesharp, there was a 51 percent reduction in at fault accidents by participants in a five-year period following the training. The American Automobile Association or AAA now offers Drivesharp at a discount to members. You may qualify you for a discount on auto insurance if you have been driving for more than 49 years, are insured by AAA, and take the Drivesharp course.

• Try the challenging and fun entertaining exercises at Brain HQ. Develop core attention, processing speed and memory by doing brain training based on science. Brain HQ recommends doing in about ninety minutes a week of online brain drills. More information is available at www. brainhq.com. Start at your own "baseline" at Luminosity and then move on to more challenging levels just like a real video game. Because Luminosity was created by both scientists and video game designers, it will increase gray matter, while you play. AARP's teamed up with the Global Council on Brain Health to create Staying Sharp, a lifestyle assessment and then bases holistic recommendations on your profile. The Staying Sharp strategies includes foods and recipes, activities, information and free brain games that will keep your mind and body healthy. To learn more visit: www.stayingsharp.com. Pushups for the brain are actually fun and rewarding.

- Garden – Almost all older adults in the Blue Zone® of Okinawa, Japan, garden. Studies of gardening demonstrate its' ability to improve mood and cognitive function. Researchers believe gardening's benefits may come from touching the earth, soil probiotics, natural light, healthy satisfaction from watching things grow as well as exercise. And I would add, gardening is good exercise and offers sensory stimulation. Pay extra attention to your sense of touch, smell, sight and taste when you garden for bonus brain stimulation.

- React in the Moment – Engage in activities that require fast reflexes such as ping pong, catch or tennis. This type of brain exercise is ideal for someone who has trouble sitting still or meditating. When you play a game that moves quickly, you are forced to pay attention. If you space out, you lose. A game of racquetball may be the perfect brain training for someone who is fast thinking, but slow to get out of their head. Games that require quick adjustments help people to connect to the physical body, yet don't require the slowing down that is needed for meditation. Reaction time typically slows as you age, and even more so if you fail to practice reacting quickly. Use it or lose its go grab a racket.

- Play Games – Chess and Bridge require working memory and reasoning skills. The Game Set (R trademark) is an excellent old school game that helps the mind practice processing. Players look for color, shape or pattern matches in the cards before their opponent. The object of the game is to beat your opponents by finding the most number of groups of same or mixed pattern matches. Set builds cognitive, logical, spatial and reasoning skills, increases processing speed and visual perception.

- Go Outside – Instead of Facebooking or Instagramming—get out of the house, go meet a friend or talk to strangers. Social Activities are incredible brain exercises that are often taken for granted. Besides having a supportive family as a predictor of a long life, another forecaster of longevity is the number of people outside of your own household you speak to any given month. Speaking to people outside of your own home reduces the risk of death. According to Claudia Kawas, professor of neurology and medicine at UC Irvine and principle researcher on the 90+ study, people don't typically don't think of interacting with acquaintances as brainwork. However according to Kawas, "People think using your brain is solving a puzzle, but when you are just getting out and interacting with people you are using your brain a lot, particularly with people you are not living with. I think you get lazy with the people you are living with. The number of times people get out of the house and interact with people outside of their family, that's cognitive exercise." You will use visual processing skills to recognize faces and short-term memory to remember new names. Small talk and questions will help with listening, processing speed and creative thinking. In studies older people who are more socially active have demonstrated an increased life expectancy. Social situations also can lift mood and alleviate feelings of depression. So, have a party, join a club or a meetup. The more you continue to learn and engage in the world, the more you grow your brain.

The Race Against Time

The amazing Ida Keeling did not begin running until she was sixty-seven years old. Grieving from the death of her two sons from drug related violence, her athletic daughter, Cheryl took her mom on a 5K run. Before the run she was grieving and depressed, "My psyche had slowed down, and it felt like I was moving around in a bowl of thick oatmeal. Not a pleasant feeling, but me and the icky sensation were becoming well acquainted. Too well." Although she struggled in that first race, she became hooked on the healing powers of running for her brain and body. She went on to set her first world record in 2008 for the 60-meter dash, ages 90–94. At age 102, she has too many world records to keep track of. In 2018, she published her memoir, *Can't Nothing Bring Me Down in the Race Against Time.* The book chronicles trace her early life In Harlem, raised by immigrant parents. She began working at age twelve. When she left home she got married had four kids and then later raised her four children as a single mother. Active in the civil rights movement she saw Malcom X speak and attended the 1963 March on Washington. "My struggles made me stronger," says Keeling. A great, great-grandmother whose athletic and inspirational feats continue to inspire the world. "I absolutely refuse to tolerate drama," Keeling writes, adding "I just don't have time for people who live only to cause trouble. Just find the nice, kind, supportive people and bring them into your circle. Let the others find God in their own way and in their own time."

- Take a day off from GPS – Drive or walk your route from memory. The hippocampus creates neurons and plays an important role in spatial navigation and organization of memory.
- Create something – Crochet, knit, paint draw, make a pottery piece. Use your hands to make things. Crafting works your fine motor skills, visual and kinesthetic sense to create. When you get crafty you will be growing and nurturing new neurons and synapses in the brain. Let go of the belief that you lack creativity. Remember that everyone is creative, and you have another opportunity to use it or lose it. In addition, if you do tend towards self-effacement, don't let your personality traits get the better of you. Never apologize for your lack of skill in anything. Keep a beginner's mind and remind yourself you may have room to improve or that you would like to improve. If you enjoy painting, drawing or crafting, never let proficiency get in your way.

- Engage in an art & learn to play a musical instrument. Or if you already play something, join a band or learn new songs. Paint, color or take a drawing class. Sign up for a flower arranging class or a singing workshop. No drug is as effective as dance says neuroscientist, Peter Davies. "The evidence says that participation in dance programs reduces the rate of development of dementia by maybe 75 percent." Playing an instrument or singing can be a particularly potent brain exercise because you will use your hearing, hand eye coordination and then your brains feedback loop to adjust to sounds you make with your voice or instrument. All that brain processing means a huge pick up in neuroplasticity.

- Brush your teeth, eat a meal or write with your nondominant hand. Using your nondominant hand will force your brain to build neurons that work a normally unused part of your brain.

- Do something new to kick your plasticity switch on. Drive a different route to work. Ride your bike to the library if you usually walk. Go to a new park once a week. Or try to do a daily or weekly activity but tell your mind that it is a new experience and treat the experience with wonder and revelation.

- Blunt one of your senses as you experience the world. Take a bite of food with your eyes closed. Smell a flower with your eyes closed. Plug your ears or turn down the volume and watch TV. Take a bath with your eyes closed. Your brain takes in information through the senses. When you block one of your senses, your brain immediately tries to make up for the lack of information and upticks the data gathering for other areas of perception.

- Read books, go to the library, or attend a lecture or book club. A Rush University Medical Center study found that lifelong readers had significantly less brain degeneration than nonreaders. Lifelong learning has been shown to decrease rates of dementia and cognitive decline.

- Play. Creative play with young children is good for your brain. Playing boosts creativity and imagination. Try a game of Charades or do some improv. Thinking on your feet and being creative in the moment builds gray matter.

IF THERE IS A WILL THERE IS A WAY

Think it's too late to go to college? In 2015, at age ninety-nine, Doreetha Daniels graduated from College of the Canyons(COC) community college in Santa Clarita, California with an associate degree in Social Sciences. She began her studies in 2009, and suffered several health setbacks along the way, including hearing and vision problems and several strokes. COC counseling faculty member, Liz Shaker was inspired by Doreetha Daniels persistence. "Doreetha is a living testament to the saying 'if there is a will, there is a way,' " COC counseling faculty member Liz Shaker said in the press release. "Her desire to get out of bed each day and come to school and face the challenges in and outside of the classroom inspired us all. She is truly an amazing woman who has impacted my life and I feel so fortunate that I was able to experience her journey alongside her." After Daniels saw several of her grandchildren enroll in graduate schools, she became inspired to go back to college. Now she advises all students. "Don't give up. Do it. Don't let anybody discourage you. Say that, 'I'm going to do it,' and do it for yourself."

Decrease the following brain deadening activities, watching TV or Netflix, iPad or iPhone. The more we engage in mindless screen time, the less we actively participate in the content entering our brain. Interaction and using senses is key to brain training. Screen time is like processed food for the brain, indulge only in moderate amounts as much as possible. And as you may know, social media and online entertainment is designed to keep you hooked. Set a timer and commit to short periods of online entertainment.

GET IN A FLOW STATE

Choose activities that engage the senses and help you to get into a flow state. Motivation is key so do things that you truly enjoy, and you can see yourself continuing to do. The one exception would be uncomfortable, but necessary growth exercises. Sometimes it is necessary to do uncomfortable things in order to learn. One example might be learning a language. When you take the time to practice learning new words and verb conjugations, when you go to Italy, you will be more prepared get into a flow state when conversing with local Italians when learning will be much more fun. There will often be uncomfortable states when learning a new skill. Super Agers know how to push through the discomfort to get to the next level. When you get into flow, you will feel satisfaction your activities and pursuits. It may take some persistence and resilience to get into a flow state.

Things You Can Do to Be Active

- Learn a language
- Take a Dance class, especially one with choreographed moves
- Golf
- Tennis
- Ping pong
- Sing
- Knit
- Crochet

- Play a musical instrument or learn a new one, piano, guitar or something more unusual
- Do a jigsaw puzzle
- Draw a map of where you live from memory
- Cook, follow a recipe
- Take a singing class, especially one that teaches you to sing more or less in key
- Go to a park or natural area and pay close attention to all of your senses; journal and draw if you can
- Go to a museum or cultural event and pay very close attention to everything; journal or draw about the event; recount to a friend everything that happened (as long as they agree and aren't bored)
- Color in a coloring book or draw or paint on blank paper

Integrating New Brain Skills

- Have a plan for integrating new brain skills into your daily schedule.
- Try something new every week.
- Take a daily walk with brain-boosting practices.
- Choose a new skill to develop and then practice daily at the same time. Examples: Create daily routines that force you to close your eyes or use your left hand or set aside time to study what you want to learn, such as dance, a language or to craft.
- Set aside weekly and monthly times to "try or do something novel."
- Seasonally travel near and far. The brain is stimulated by your environment so travel in your area or book a trip to a foreign country, your brain will reap the benefits!
- Don't force yourself to do all the hard stuff at once. Remember motivation has importance. If you aren't ready to change your ways, acknowledge it and either wait until you are ready or come up with a plan to take baby steps.

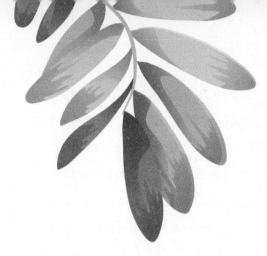

CHAPTER 11

Super Ager Meditation

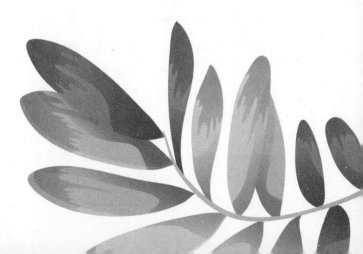

"*Dr. Walsh then listed eight lifestyle factors that have been shown to contribute to healthy aging. These include exercise, diet, time in nature, relationships, recreation, stress management, and service to others. As soon as I saw this list I realized that a spiritual approach to aging and modern research had a lot in common. And when I read the last factor-religious and spiritual involvement-I was sure of it. Ancient Taoists and Buddhists combined meditation, exercise, diet, herbs, and minerals to support long life. Clearly, they were on to something! Modern research points us in the same direction.*"

—Lewis Richmond, *Aging as a Spiritual Practice: A Contemplative Guide to Growing Older and Wiser*

LIVE IN THE AGELESS ZONE WITH MEDITATION

Meditation is one of the simplest actions that you can add to your aging toolkit. Meditation costs nothing, can be done, almost anywhere and has so many benefits. Although it can be challenging for some to sit still. Fortunately, there are numerous work arounds if you have never tried it or are generally more distractible. To help you get over the challenges of beginning a meditation practice. The rewards and results are many, meditation supports mental, emotional and physical health at little or no cost. In a fast paced, stressed out world, meditation can be one the most important "go-to" remedies for aging.

Holding Still

Mary Sullivan, scientist, Ayurveda practitioner and yoga therapist experienced a health crisis on a road trip with her husband. "As a scientist who integrates, Ayurveda, yoga and medicine in my life, emergency health issues or systems failures head me straight to western medicine, where I know I will get fast symptom treatment and system & tissue repair. I advise my clients to do the same." Yet Mary also carries Ayurveda wisdom into any illness or health crisis. "In the middle of nowhere in New Mexico, a few years ago, on vacation, I had a serious eye problem. I looked over at my husband and said, 'I can't see out of my left eye anymore.' " Instead of a view there was a gray river, which turned out, was blood. Mary and her husband headed straight to the nearest medical center, not an Ayurvedic practitioner. As she sat in the ER waiting room, waiting, she meditated. Once I was seen, the ER doc looked in her eye and said, "Wow I can't see anything." "Neither can I," she replied and continued meditating. A specialist was called in who sent her to a bigger hospital. The problem turned out to be a detached retina with lots of bleeding in the eye.

At the hospital she was given three choices, lose the sight in her eye, have an operation on site and consequently hang out in Arizona for up to six months to heal or head home immediately for care. The Boston area where Mary lived has some of the best eye surgeons in the United States. Off she went eastbound on the next plane and into surgery that very day. She used meditation and pranayama (breathing) to still her mind and relax on her flight home. Quietly she chanted quietly during her operation until the doctor said, "This is the delicate part I need you to be quiet and hold really still." Who knew that "hold still" would be a key part of her recovery? She had to hold her head at a precise angle twenty-three hours a day for about three months for the operation to succeed. She couldn't read or watch TV. Instead she meditated multiple times each day and listened to books on tape. Before, during and after her operation she used mind-body healing techniques from *Prepare for Surgery Heal Faster* by Peggy Huddleston to boost her recovery. Mantra, or the repetition of key phrases was also an essential part of her healing process. After recovering from the operation, she contacted a natural vision coach, upped her daily eye care, worked on balancing the heat in her eyes and used yoga therapy to help my neck muscles loosen up and recover. Now fully recovered, Mary Sullivan feels eternally grateful for the contemplative practices that sustained her and got her through a health crisis that required her not to move for twenty-three hours a day for three months-amazing!

Thirty meditators went to Shambhala mountain in northern Colorado for a three-month retreat. Participants meditated for six hours a day for the entire three months. Their telomere length and function were evaluated before and after the retreat. The results were astonishing. The meditators had a 30 percent increase in telomerase activity, the enzyme that increases and protects telomeres. And the study also found that those that meditated had an increased sense of purpose, and less negative emotions compared to a control group who came to the mountain but did not meditate. Meditation may boost life expectancy by up to 30 percent based on the findings of this study.

There are many types of meditation and without comparing and contrasting all of the variety of meditation techniques. Here are a few to try. Most notable is simple mindful breath awareness.

Nobel laureate and scientist, Elizabeth Blackburn reminds us we can renew our telomeres and our cells, *right now!* Her book, co-authored with Elisa Epel, *The Telomere Effect*, contains many useful and helpful tips based on research of telomeres. Longer telomeres are associated with longer life expectancy. One study showed that people who focus on the activity that they are currently engaged in, had longer telomeres than those whose minds tend to wander more. Other studies demonstrated the power of mindfulness training and meditation for improved telomere maintenance. Blackburn stresses that because mental focus is a skill that can be developed, it should not be overlooked as an important tool for mental and physical health.

MINDFULNESS MEDITATION

Sit comfortably, with a long spine in a quiet place. Set a specific amount of time to practice. It is recommended that you use a timer or set an alarm. Otherwise you may be distracted by a need to check the time. If you are new to meditation, start with a very short meditation, even one to three minutes for at least a week is great. Then work up to five, then ten, fifteen minutes, twenty minutes, half an hour. Meditating for twenty to thirty minutes a day is a big accomplishment.

In mindfulness meditation you simply focus on your breath. Rest your hands on your lap, close your eyes or lower your gaze with your eyes open. Relax your mind and body and then begin focusing on the breath. It may help to focus on a particular sensation such as the air entering your nostrils. Keep following the breath until the next thing that happens. You will become distracted, you will day dream or think about something else. You won't be thinking about your breath. So, the moment you notice when this happens, simply bring your attention and awareness back to the breath. Keep doing these three steps:

1. Focus on your breath.
2. Notice when your mind wanders.
3. Come back to your focus on the breath.

Repeat these steps ad infinitum. If you find it impossible to focus on your breath, don't fight it. Let your mind wander. Eventually your mind will simmer down, almost like a pot that is boiling over. Eventually the mind will cool, and the bubbling water will settle to stillness.

A Worldly Woman

Indra Devi was a Russian yoga teacher who was born in 1899. She first read a book about yoga as a when she was fifteen years old. In 1927, she boarded a boat and headed for India where she became an actress and later studied yoga with legendary, T. Krishnamacharya who at the time did not take female students, especially western women. She lived and taught yoga all over the world, establishing yoga schools in China, the United States, Mexico and Buenos Aires. She taught Richard Hittleman, another early American yoga author and teacher. She herself authored several books on yoga, including the first yoga book written by a westerner and published in India and the popular, *Yoga for Americans*. In the 1950s, she taught yoga to Hollywood celebrities including Gloria Swanson, Eva Gabor and Greta Garbo. She moved to Argentina in 1985, where she lived until her death at 102 years old.

DIVINE PURPOSE MEDITATION

We know that meditation helps people feel like they are connected with purpose. This meditation is designed to accelerate a meditative connection to your purpose so that as you age you feel in communion with your own purpose, dharma and reason for living. See Chapter 2 for more information on how purpose has been associated with a longer life. Sit tall, with a long spine on a cushion or in a chair. Begin by placing one hand on your heart center, right in the center of your chest on your sternum. Connect to the feeling in your heart, feel your heart beating and the movement of your breath. Notice feelings and sensations. Keep connecting without judgment, even if sadness, anger or any other uncomfortable emotions arise. Don't push any emotions away. If you haven't connected to your own heart in a long time or if you tend to be someone who focuses on others rather than yourself, this focused action may be uncomfortable. Keep going though, the harder this meditation is for you, the more powerful the results. If you like to focus on others and not yourself, you will find this to be a powerful meditation. And the counterintuitive thing about helping others, but not yourself. You will be healthier and better at helping others once you learn to focus on your own heart center.

After one to five minutes, place your other hand around your navel in the center or your body. Feel your belly. What do you notice, again be aware of feelings and or sensations? Do you feel uncomfortable, judgmental, full of regret or sadness? Don't push those feelings away. Next breathe low in your body and feel like your energy is going low. Imagine your breath filling your pelvic bowl. If you are feeling sadness or heavy emotions. Keep feeling and breathing. Return to this meditation daily. When you feel light in this meditation which could be on day one or day ten or day thirty. If it takes longer than thirty days to feel emotionally light, check with your doctor or other practitioner. Think of a feeling of joy. If it is hard to feel joy, think of a pet, a baby or someone that sparks true unconditional love in you. Meditate on this feeling for five to twenty minutes. Feel and sense this joy; imagine: If it were a color, what color would it be? Bring this color all around you breathe it into every cell. Then at the same sitting or at another time. Bring up this color and feeling of joy. Start to think of the activities big and small that bring you this same unconditional love and joy. Write them down. Keep meditating on this feeling of joy.

Next phase, after doing your Divine Purpose Meditation. Grab your journal and write your divine purpose. What words resonate for you if not purpose? Ikigai? Dharma, reason for living or reason for being? What would you like to contribute to the world Is it a color or can you describe it? Is it evolving. Most important in your purpose is it fills you with joy. So, ask yourself the question, what brings me joy? Then write about it.

Metta Meditation

This meditation is also known as loving kindness meditation. Practice this meditation when you feel internalized criticism or ageist beliefs that you have taken on. Metta is first practiced on yourself. Often it is difficult to feel or cultivate self-love. Begin by sitting quietly, taking relaxed, slow, deep breaths and wishing yourself happiness. After sitting quietly begin to say these words silently or on occasion out loud to yourself. "May I be happy. May I be well. May I be safe. May I be peaceful and at ease." Continue this practice until you feel "full" of self-love and compassion. If you have difficulty raising up a sense of self-love. Think of a baby or a beloved pet to help evoke the sentiment of pure unconditional love. When you are ready to move to the next phase, begin to think of another person you would like to give happiness and unconditional love to. Send the love through your meditation and saying these words, "May you be happy. May you be well. May you be safe. May you be peaceful and at ease." After the first person, you can focus your thoughts on a group or another person and go through the same process. You can choose your family or the people in your city or even the citizens of the world. This meditation increases self-love, the ability to love unconditionally as well as greater connection to others.

NOISE AND STRESS

In the mid-twentieth century, epidemiologists discovered a link between high blood pressure, tinnitus, sleep loss, heart disease and chronic noise sources. People who worked in noisy environments such as automotive parts manufacturing plant or at a mall were found to have increases in blood pressure and heart rates. Other studies linked high blood pressure and heart disease with living in close proximity to a noisy airport. As researchers discovered too much noise lead to stress, tension, and health decline, they consequently detected silence can release chronic tension and relax the body and brain. In a 2006 study done by Luciano Bernardi, the benefits of silence were tested against the effects of music. Researchers monitored physiological markers for two dozen test subjects while they listened to six musical tracks. The effect music had on the subjects could be detected via changes in blood pressure, carbon dioxide, and circulation in the brain. The findings made sense, given that active listening requires attention. But Bernardi accidentally found that randomly added silence between songs had also an effect. The two-minute silent pauses proved far more relaxing than music or a longer silence played before the experiment started. In another study, four groups of mice were subjected to different sounds, either white noise, music, calls of baby mice or silence. Guess what? The mice whose brains were bathed in silence generated a surge in new neurons, indicating that silence holds great promise for brain health and neuroplasticity. Meditators have been found to have faster brain processing speeds and significantly greater amounts of gray matter. Dr. Dale Bredesen routinely recommends meditation for his Alzheimer's patients and remarks that as a science based, medical doctor never thought that if you told him just a few years ago that he would have recommended something like meditation to his patients, he would not have believed it.

The strain of modern day life, the constant divided attention, high tension situations—put pressure on our prefrontal cortex brain (which is responsible for problem-solving, high order thinking and decision-making). Thanks to Attention Restoration Study we now know we can restore the brain's cognitive resources and regenerate brain cells by placing ourselves in environments with lower sensory input, like sitting in silence or taking a walk in nature.

T. Krishnamarcharya, 1888–1989

Krishnamarcharya lived to be 100 years of age and is credited with founding modern yoga because of his extensive knowledge and the high-profile yoga teachers he taught and influenced. He held six Vedic degrees, the equivalent of six PhDs in subjects of law, Ayurvedic medicine, logic and others. In India he was known as a healer who used both Ayurveda and yoga to restore health to those he treated. From 1926–46 he ran a yoga school for young boys in Mysore. He taught and influenced, K. Patabbhi Jois, the founder of Ashtanga yoga, his brother in law, BKS Iyengar, founder of Iyengar yoga, his son, TKV Desikachar, founder of Viniyoga, AG Mohan, founder of Svastha yoga and Indra Devi, a Russian yoga teacher and author, who brought yoga around the world. Krishnamacharya promoted yoga practice through his demonstrations of the practice and travel throughout India. His demos sometimes included siddhis, or supernatural powers of yoga such as suspending his pulse and the lifting of extremely heavy objects or the stopping of the movement of a car for example. He also performed difficult advanced asanas or yoga poses to garner attention for the practice. He was known for performing a detailed intake of all patients and yoga students that included pulse diagnosis, observation of the quality of a person's skin and breath as well as other pertinent health questions. He would also ascertain whether a person would be willing to follow his instructions, which often included not only yoga instructions, but, herbal medicines, breathing practices, meditations and dietary adjustments. Krishnamacharya "believed yoga to be India's greatest gift to the world." and approached each person and student as unique, knowing that the path of yoga and healing was never one-size-fits-all. During meditation he respected all religious or nonreligious beliefs. He instructed students to close their eyes and, "think of God, if not God, the sun. If not the sun, your parents."

LIVE AN UNHURRIED LIFE MEDITATION

This meditation is helpful when feeling overwhelmed by circumstances and or when you have a deadline and feel as though you have too much to do. Often, we may "speed up" to get more done. Yet speeding up without focus and multitasking are often if not always counterproductive. The meditation derives its name from residents of the Ogimi village in Okinawa who are known for longevity. One of their shared values is, "live an unhurried life." This can be done as a seated meditation or as a walking meditation.

Seated Meditation

Sit tall on a cushion or in a chair. Take off your shoes and or your socks if you can. If you are on a chair feel the soles of your feet where your arches are located. Feel for feet and then imagine that your feet have little vacuums or suction cups in the arches. Allow the arches of your feet to become portals for the earth energy to rise and travel up your legs, through your calves, knee joints and then your thighs. In this meditation it might be helpful to imagine that you are like a living geyser or a fountain. A geyser pulls up water from deep in the earth and then shoots it out. You are going to imagine you are pulling up the earth in a liquid form, imagine water if that is helpful. Pull it up through your legs and then let it pool at the base of your spine. Next let it flow back down into the earth like a waterfall. Take five to ten minutes and just follow this flow of energy downward and back into the earth. Let this energy flow back into the ground taking with it any rushing. The earth and nature naturally slow us down. Just keep feeling the slow flow. Finally let the energy build and start to fountain out through your spine and sushumna nadi. As the energy moves up like a geyser, let it fountain out through the top of your head. Let it clean out the area around your body and your aura. Let it also clean out your body, like a shower. Let this shower of earth vibration clean out your body and energy field for about five to ten minutes. At the end take a few deep breaths and notice if you feel like things have slowed down.

Walking Meditation

To do this meditation while walking. Walk slowly and rhythmically feeling your body in space. Notice the arches of your feet. Feel sensations arising from the arches of your feet. You can focus on the instep or to take this meditation one step further, feel as though you are pulling up the earth into your body as you walk. Each time your foot hits the ground, imagine a magnetic pull that draws up the electron force of the planet into your body. You could do this practice barefoot for added benefit or just end by taking off your shoes and taking 1–5 minutes breathing barefoot with your feet on the ground.

-PRACTICE PLAN-

Meditation Habits

As a daily habit, spend one to thirty minutes meditating. Use an app or one of the above listed meditations. Read *Aging as a Spiritual Practice* by Lewis Redmond and try some of his excellent meditations. It is also available on Audible.

Daily Habits

- Meditate at the same time daily. Try meditating in the morning after you wake up or after your morning tea or coffee. Try it at your lunch break or when you get home from work. Or maybe your best shot would be a before bed meditation.

- Remember to start small. If you have never meditated before, make your meditation so easy and so short, you can't say no. Start with one minute, work up to five, then maybe ten or thirty minutes or even longer. If it helps use an app, there are many good ones you can download Headspace, 10 Percent Happier, Calm or Smiling Minds. All have free trials and then a nominal monthly fee. Smiling Minds, however is always free.

- Go to www.10percenthappier.com for a fun, innovative, down to earth approach to meditation.

Weekly Habits

- Meditate in nature, take a walk in nature. Every week, plan a special mindful walk in nature when you have extra time, perhaps on the weekend or in the evening.

- Sign up for a meditation class or go to a meditation group.

- Form your own group of likeminded peers and meditate on your own or hire a teacher to guide the group.

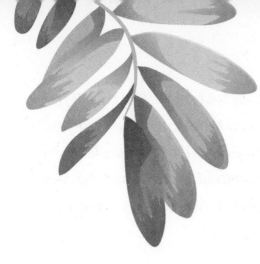

CHAPTER 12

Natural Medicines to Boost Body, Mind, and Spirit at Any Age

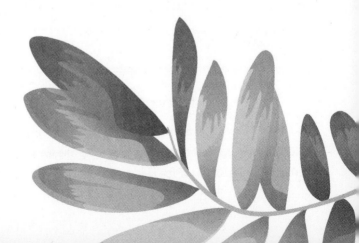

"We have finally started to notice that there is real curative value in local herbs and remedies. In fact, we are also becoming aware that there are little or no side effects to most natural remedies, and that they are often more effective than Western medicine."

—Anne Wilson Schaef

Before modern medicine, humans relied on plants and natural substances for their medicine. Phytotherapy describes the branch of pharmacology that deals with using plants to heal by making infusions, decoctions, herbal teas and extracts. The Greeks had their own version of Ayurveda where the five elements, seasons, and qualities governed medicines and life-force cycles. Herbal medicine has always been a part of Ayurveda and traditional Chinese medicine. On the island of Ikaria, Greece, islanders drink plenty of mountain tea and herbal brews of wild rosemary, sage and oregano. These diuretic teas keep blood pressure low and increase tea drinkers' antioxidant levels. Many traditional healing systems rely on teas and herbal medicine to support healthy aging and prevent disease.

Natural Remedies

Bhagavan Kani, 115 years old, is a spiritual leader. He lives in the Spice Mountains and is a member of the Kani people who live in the region above Kerala, India. Although his age remains "unverified," because at the date of his birth, written records did not exist in his tribe. Local leaders and family members can verify his age. He gatherers fruits and vegetables for his own meals daily. Occasionally someone from his large extended family brings him a prepared meal. He walks in nature with two large walking sticks, collecting interesting objects he finds along the way that he makes into garlands and more walking sticks. For his daily routine, he rises before dawn, watches the sunrise and drinks tulsi tea followed by a light breakfast of raw fruits and vegetables. Later he enjoys time with the youngest members of his family, often recounting tales of his own childhood. In the afternoon he walks to a nearby hill where he says prayers and makes offerings to deities, singing and talking to plants and animals. He is the head healer of his community, using leaves, roots, bark and plants in rituals to heal various ailments. His memory is sharp, and he climbs hills with ease.

Natural medicines especially teas, medicinal drinks and pastes have been a part of healing traditions around the world for thousands of years. This chapter will focus on the simplicity of natural medicine. Check with your own Integrative Physician, medical doctor, licensed acupuncturist, Naturopathic doctor, or Functional Medicine doctor for a personalized list of natural medicines and supplements that would serve you and your healthy aging.

Teas: As you age your sense of thirst declines and has an inverse effect, the more dehydrated you are, the less you want to drink. Having a habit of drinking tea, is rather than coffee or alcohol can be especially beneficial and one of the best reasons to drink tea as the years roll. Caffeinated teas do contain of course caffeine, so use in moderation and mix with other, herbal teas or drinks.

How the Thirst Sensors in the Brain Decline with Age

Dehydration occurs when your body doesn't have enough water and other fluids to function normally. Dehydration can happen to anyone, but it is more persistent and more common in older adults. Our bodies lose water every day when we breathe, perspire, urinate, and have bowel movements. As we age, our sense of thirst decreases, and the kidneys aren't able to conserve body water as well. Over the age of fifty, you may start to feel tired rather than thirsty and may opt for a nap instead of the liquid your body needs. If you remain dehydrated, you can end up suffering complications, some of which can be severe.

Why does lack of thirst and the resulting dehydration increase as we get older? A study was done in 2001 that dealt with the subject of "Influence of age thirst and fluid intake." It was discovered that even though older adults (over sixty-five years old) consume sufficient volumes of fluids on a daily basis, when challenged by fluid deprivation/dehydration or exercise in a warmer environment, the older adults experience decreased thirst sensation and reduced fluid intake. Exercise in a warmer environment caused dehydration, and those in the study did not feel the urge to hydrate in congruity with the amount of liquid that was needed by their bodies. Their bodies came up short in the short-term, because of their dulled thirst signals. The study concluded that the aging process impairs physiological control systems which are associated with thirst and satiety.

One study compared men in their twenties to those in their sixties. Both were injected with a saline solution that would create a need for water. Young and older men all felt thirsty after the injection, yet the older men drank only half the amount of water as their twenty-year-old counterparts. PET scans revealed that there was less activity in the brains of the men in their sixties as they gulped water to quench their thirst. Researchers believe that nerves that send a thirsty signal to the brain become less effective as we age. And ironically, probably the more older adults ignore our weak thirst signals, the more the brain and body become dehydrated further decreasing the brains cries for hydration. One of the simplest ways to combat the decreased thirst impulse that occurs with age is to make it a daily habit to hydrate first thing in the morning. Ayurveda recommends a glass of warm water with lemon. Drink 12–24 ounces of water every morning. Add lemon for an extra cleansing and alkalizing effect.

Teas have a long history in many cultures of fortifying health and longevity. The first tea was said to have been made when a leaf floated off of a tree into a cup of hot water in China.

Listed below are some important teas, herbal and caffeinated that are beneficial to your health and that will promote healthy aging. In Ayurveda, drinking hot or warm water is most beneficial because warm or hot water does not cool digestive fire. Many Americans habitually drink iced drinks or store water and other drinks in the refrigerator. Try drinking water at room temperature or heat it. In Ayurveda warm or hot water helps to clear ama or toxins from the body.

- **Green Tea** – In recent decades, green tea has been studied extensively for its antioxidant properties. Green tea is loaded with polyphenols like flavonoids and catechins. One powerful compound present in green tea is Epigallocatechin Gallate, L-Theanine increases activity of the anti-anxiety neurotransmitter GABA. Green tea has been shown to boost metabolic rate and reduce risk of Alzheimer's and Parkinson's disease. An eleven-year study of 40,000 Japanese study participants found that those that drank more green tea were less likely to die, especially from cardiovascular disease.

- **Oolong Tea** – Oolong tea is partially fermented black tea. Both oolong tea and green tea have been shown to boost metabolism. Oolong tea contains more caffeine than green tea, but less than black tea. As a traditional Chinese beverage, oolong tea has been known to support weight loss in Asian cultures. Science is now beginning to validate that claim. One study showed that polyphenols exclusive to oolong tea can help you lose weight. The study concluded that indeed oolong tea, "could decrease body fat content and reduce body weight through improved lipid metabolism."

- **White Tea** – Highest in antioxidants and lowest in caffeine, white tea is brewed at a low temperature. It has a mild flavor which blends well with herbal ingredients. Many people prefer to drink white tea it without accompanying ingredients, however white tea is often blended with other medicinal herbs because of its mild flavor.

- Pu-erh Tea-Traditionally consumed after meals in China to help with digestion. Pu-erh tea is uniquely processed and often aged. Pu-erh has less antioxidants than other types of tea and has not been studied as extensively.

- **Black Tea** – Drink the tea you enjoy the most and if that tea is black tea there will be many health benefits. Black tea contains catechins and has more concentrated amounts of the powerful antioxidant flavonoids, thearubigins and theaflavin. Growing evidence suggests that black tea has some of the anti-cancer properties that green tea contains. Several studies have shown that tannins in black tea help fight viruses such as influenza, dysentery and hepatitis.

- **Kombucha Tea** – and probiotics combined sounds like a great longevity blend, however kombucha tea has not been studied as much as other traditional teas. Kombucha has found favor in health food circles because of its taste and anecdotal health benefits. It has some caffeine and a little alcohol. In Ayurveda, Kombucha has a sour flavor which does not go well with fire. If you are fifty-plus, the flavor and properties of Kombucha may be beneficial according to Ayurveda because you will need more fire and digestive power as you age. Check with your own health care professional if you aren't sure Kombucha is for you.

- **Rooibos** – An excellent alternative to caffeinated teas, this high in antioxidant tea blends well with other herbs to make a tea. See Rooibos chai below

- **Ginger Tea** – Cut up one or two one-inch pieces of ginger and then boil these chunks of ginger in about sixteen to twenty-four ounces of water. Note the water will decrease and you can double or triple this recipe and keep this healing tea on hand. Ayurveda reveres ginger as a universal healer and it is among the healthiest herbs on the planet. A root, ginger is good for all types of people and all stages of life. It can also be consumed in powdered form. Tea bags may also contain dried pieces of ginger. Gingerol the main compound in ginger has powerful anti-inflammatory and antioxidant properties. Ginger's anti-inflammatory properties may help decrease pain and need for medication in those that suffer from osteoarthritis. Ginger has been shown to lower blood sugar and cardiovascular risks in diabetics. Ginger traditionally has been used to support digestion and scientific studies have demonstrated that ginger appears to speed up the rate at which the stomach empties implicating its impact on healthy digestion. Some evidence suggests ginger may reduce bad cholesterol in animals and humans. More studies are needed, but ginger seems to have cancer protective properties.

- **Chai** – The word chai means tea, so when most people say chai, they are referring to Masala chai, a spicy black tea served with milk and sweetener. There are many variations of chai spices. A few are essential and can be added fresh or dried. Chai spices support physical energy and digestion. The fresher the herbs, the more potent the healing potential of Masala chai. Cardamom, ginger, black pepper, cloves, cinnamon, star anise. Aging can make you more sensitive to caffeine and many types of premade chai or those purchased in a restaurant or cafe can be quite high in caffeine. It is possible to buy chai tea in tea bags, but these usually are not in the same league with homemade chai. Make your own decaf version with rooibos. See recipe below.

Age-Slowing Rooibos Chai

- (Use dry, powdered herbs)
- ½ cup Rooibos
- ½ ground cardamom
- ½ cup of ground cinnamon
- ½ cup of ground ginger
- 2 TBSP. ground Turmeric
- 2 TBSP. ground cloves,
- 2 tsps. of ground pepper
- Add honey and milk (vegan milk or other milks) to taste

CCF Tea

- **Lemon Balm** – a member of the mint family, Paracelsus, a well-known sixteenth-century Swiss herbalist referred to lemon balm as an "elixir of life." He noted that lemon balm helps to build strength and increase longevity. Lemon Balm has a long history in European folk medicine as a memory enhancer and is currently being investigated as an herb for treating Alzheimer's or creating a new drug based on lemon balm active compounds.

   Recent studies on lemon balm demonstrate the herb's ability to support secondary memory and the ability to learn. Current science behind lemon balm indicates that it may have some preventative effects for Alzheimer's disease.

- **Tulsi Tea** – Ganesh the elephant headed Indian god wears a garland of tulsi leaves around his neck as an auspicious symbol. Tulsi is an adaptogen, meaning you can never have too much of it. The more tulsi you drink or consume, the more benefits you will receive and there are many. Tulsi tea helps your body mitigate stress and builds immunity. You can buy tulsi as a supplement or tea. Loaded with antioxidants, the herb can regulate blood sugar and ward off the common cold.

- **Mint** – Fresh or dried mint leaf tea offers many benefits to those who drink it. Grow a mint plant on your counter or in your yard and you will always have a source of fresh delicious mint for tea and other dishes. Mint calms a queasy tummy. It activates salivary glands, treats nausea and headache. It also helps to clear congestion and treat asthma. It can also be used as an essential oil which is good for reducing depression and treating fatigue.

She Has Something to Brag About: Patricia Bragg

Wearing her signature pink straw hat with roses, strands of big pearls and a 100-watt smile, fifth generation Californian, Patricia Bragg has been extolling the virtues of a healthy organic lifestyle long before it was ever in vogue. She never gives her age because her beliefs seem more connected to the infinite. "I don't believe in age. I feel ageless and believe in eternity. In my heart, I feel eighteen, If I said "eighteen," you would think that was ridiculous. I don't have an ache or pain and I have no stiffness. Age is just in our head." After a good night's sleep, she does her deep breathing exercises, then jogs in place for five minutes, followed by windmill ab work. An advocate of dry-brushing and morning smoothies, she takes regular barefoot walks in nature. Always a trendsetter, she's been going shoeless, before earthing was a thing. Her adopted father, Paul C Bragg opened up the first health food store in Los Angeles and traveled the country spreading the word about health food and healthy living. As LA and Hollywood grew so did health food and the Bragg empire. Known as health guru to the stars, Patricia Bragg runs Braggs Live Foods, a company established in 1912, and now based in Santa Barbara. Braggs distributes olive oil, apple cider vinegar, instructional books and spice mixes to Whole Foods, health-oriented grocers and to customers worldwide through an online store. As for Patricia, she says her diet consists of 80 percent organic fruits, vegetables and legumes. She fuels her youthful exuberance with sweet potatoes, lentils and fresh soup are on her greatest hits list. As a pioneer and uber successful health food business woman, Patricia Braggs travels the world spreading her wisdom. When she is at home she enjoys nature, her rose garden and gathering her own honey. Gwyneth Paltrow, the Dalai Lama and Katy Perry season meals with salt-free, gluten-free, and vegan Braggs aminos. A proponent of fasting, Patricia takes time off: "Every religion has a period of fasting and it's been used to heal the sick. When you use it correctly, fasting can help reverse the aging process." A wise old soul she is.

Recipe for Bragg's Apple Cider Vinegar Lemon and Honey Drink

Benefits include, increases potassium, decreases muscle cramps, antibacterial properties, reduces inflammation, balances stomach acid, stimulates enzymes, lowers blood pressure and cholesterol. Honey boosts energy and a study in Japan found that apple cider vinegar reduced body fat and waistlines in obese people. Buy Organic Braggs Apple Cider Vinegar Drink all natural or make your own, using recipe below.

- Glass of water (hot, cold or room temperature) 12-16 ounces of water
- 2 tablespoons Braggs Apple Cider Vinegar

- 2 tablespoons Lemon Juice
- 1–3 teaspoons raw honey
- Optional ½–1 teaspoon ground ginger

- **Chamomile** – I often serve chamomile tea to my restorative yoga students. I choose organic or wildcrafted chamomile and brew it strong. Everyone gasps because they aren't used to such delicious chamomile tea as it is often served as a strong brew how. Don't settle for mediocre chamomile. This calming medicinal herb contains so many potent phytochemicals and it tastes delicious too, when you source it well and brew it strong.

- **Rosehips** – Use crushed or dried rosehips to make a delicious and healthy tea. Rosehip tea combines well with hibiscus flowers and together will lower blood sugar and boost immunity. Rosehips are very high in antioxidants, flavonoids, and vitamin C. It also increases metabolic function and detoxifies the body by increasing metabolism. Reduce inflammation and lower risk of heart disease by drinking rosehip tea.

- **Nettle Tea** – Use tea bags or dried leaves. Nettle, also known as *urtica dioica* in Latin, has been used for thousands of years as a powerful medicinal tea. Nettle leaves are extremely rich in minerals and most commonly used to treat urinary problems, urinary tract infections, and allergies. Nettle consists of flavonoids, vitamin C and B, sterols and minerals. When brewed as a tea, nettle leaves are a rich source of easily absorbed magnesium, which making the tea fantastic immune system booster, as well as a drink to calm your mind and body. Try nettle tea before you reach for antihistamines, it helps to clear allergies. As a diuretic, it also has a positive effect on kidneys and it improves urinary flow. Nettle tea also can prevent kidney stones. Because it's rich in calcium, magnesium, and iron, nettle tea is an excellent choice for older adults and people at risk for osteoporosis. With age, the mineral density of our bones decreases and drinking nettle tea is a quick and easy way to nourish our bodies with more antioxidants and minerals. In a study done by the University of Frankfurt, people with arthritis reported relieved pain while using a combination of anti-inflammatory medications and stewed nettles. Studies have also shown a positive effect of nettle on blood pressure in animals, though this still has to be shown on humans. Nettle tea shouldn't be taken by people with heart disease or kidney problems. And strongly brewed nettle tea can also interact with some other medicines and over-the-counter medications, so it's always best to check in with your doctor.

- **Fennel Tea** – A traditional tea in China, India and the Middle East. Fennel tea can be made with the seeds, leaves or the bulb. Fennel contains estrogen like compounds and is helpful in reducing the symptoms of menopause or perimenopause. Fennel tea stimulates digestion and reduces inflammation. Fennel tea helps reduce inflammation and for this reason it can soothe sore, inflamed gums. Because it naturally detoxifies the body as well as reduces inflammation, fennel tea reduces pain from gout and arthritis. It can help tone skin because of its estrogenic and anti-inflammatory properties. Drink fennel tea when you have a cold or to reduce symptoms of asthma, fennel has antimicrobial properties.

- **Triphala** – A traditional herbal Ayurvedic formula made with three fruits, including Amalki or Indian gooseberry. Triphala has been used in Indian medicines for thousands of years. It's safe for all people, especially older people, triphala is often used therapeutically for gastrointestinal issues. Triphala has been studied extensively in India and the west. Research has demonstrated the efficacy of triphala for numerous health conditions. Triphala extract was shown to significantly reduce free radical activity, considered a major factor in aging. Triphala protected against stress induced behavioral alterations, as well as several other types of stress in animal studies. Western Medicine is coming to the conclusion that much of our health comes from the gut, something that was always a given in Ayurveda. Triphala main use in Ayurveda was to support digestion. Triphala acts as a mild laxative and supports healthy gut bacteria, such as triphala research suggests that it can be helpful in treating colitis. Polyphenols present in triphala promote a healthy intestinal microbiome by supporting healthy bacteria such as bifidobacteria and lactobacillus, while inhibiting unhealthy gut bacteria.

Hormones are the body's natural messengers. They play a vital role in almost every function of our body. Hormone health is foundational to healthy aging. A healthy endocrine system functions like a symphony. All endocrine organs function together to produce a melody of hormones that work together to insure good health. Hormones naturally decline with age, yet with natural support, you will retain good hormonal function as you age. In Okinawa, Japan men and women generally have much higher hormone levels than American counterparts of the same age. If you suffer from insomnia, low sex drive, mood swings, depression, excessive hot flashes or weight gain during perimenopause, chances are you may need help balancing your hormones. Consult with your primary care physician, Licensed acupuncturist, Functional Medicine doctor for treatment. For general hormonal support supplements that balance and boost hormones as one ages are listed below:

- **Maca** – This root was used by ancient shamans of Peru. Grown in the high elevation of mountains of the Andes where many plants can't survive, maca was taken by warriors to improve their stamina in battle. As a natural adaptogen, maca has a long history of boosting both men and women's libido. Maca is an ideal herb for the endocrine system as it will naturally boost under producing glands, while it inhibits over production in glands that are out of balance and producing extra hormones. Maca root is available in powder form so you can add it to smoothies, water or juice. Or you can take it as a tablet or capsule to balance the thyroid, thymus, pancreas, pituitary gland, hypothalamus, ovaries or gonads.

- **Ashwagandha** – Many older adults complain about having fatigue and having difficulty being able to relax. Enter Ashwagandha, an Ayurveda super herb, that helps to energize you and calm you down all at the same time. Known to supports a healthy nervous system, Ashwagandha is good for sleep, inducing calm and reproductive function. Physician Dr. Dale Bredesen, author of, *The End of Alzheimer's*, uses Ashwagandha as a part of his Alzheimer healing protocol, he calls ReCODE. For more information on Dr. Bredesen and his protocol, go here, https://www. drbredesen.com/protocoloverview Ashwagandha supports thyroid and adrenal health and helps to sustain energy, especially for adults who are under stress or undergoing strenuous athletic activity.

MINDFUL MENOPAUSE

As women age, estrogen declines and ovary function declines, perimenopause begins. The trouble is that the transition to menopause when the ovaries cease to function occurs gradually over time, so perimenopause can be difficult to pinpoint. And perimenopause is when most women have what are considered menopausal symptoms, such as hot flashes, weight gain, mood swing, insomnia and lack of sex drive. Can you be symptom free during perimenopause. Ayurveda expert and Yoga Health Coach, Alexandra Epple says yes! According to her menopause is the shift from the Pitta stage of life to the Vata stage of life for women. Ayurveda doesn't really talk about menopause, but instead considers each woman as unique, and from that vantage point strives to help each woman go through perimenopause as smoothly as possible depending on her circumstances.

According to Alexandra Epple, there are three types of menopause which correlate with the different mind-body-spirit types of Ayurveda. If you are more of a Vata or air type, you will experience more dryness and anxiety during your transition to menopause. If you have more of a Pitta constitution you will have lots more hot flashes and inflammation. Not fun, but good to know. And if you are more of a steady Kapha type, you will luckily be less symptomatic, but possible have more weight gain.

Here are Alexandra Epple's quick fixes for hot flashes:

1. Avoid alcohol, caffeine, and junk food to minimize bursts of extreme heat and sweating that occur during hot flashes. If you have had hot flashes, you may consider it worth it to make these changes, even if only temporarily.

2. Carry a shawl. Your body is in transition, so be prepared for your own microclimate independent of others in the room, or outdoors, when your body is moving into this new stage, make yourself comfortable and because you never know when you may be hot or cold.

3. Embrace the hot flash. It may sound slightly silly, but the more you fight them, the more they can aggravate you. When you feel a hot flash coming on, think of welcoming the heat or leaning in to experience all your body's communication. Tell someone that you are having a hot flash. Believe it or not it helps.

According to Dr. Christiane Northrup, menopause presents an opportunity. During this time, known as the change, you any undigested toxins or experiences will return to you stronger than ever. In other words, trauma, old wounds and physical ailments that you never treated will get worse during perimenopause and menopause. The gift is that if there is anything you unknowingly and unwittingly pushed away or suppressed, you get to revisit and heal once and for all. The transition to menopause is a time to nourish yourself, relax, meditate and rejuvenate. It is not a disease and symptoms are optional according to Alexandra Epple. Learn more about Alexandra Epple, her work and her podcast, "Women Gone Vibrant" at www.alexandraepple.com. Also check out Dr. Christiane Northrup at www.drnorthrup.com or find her book, *The Wisdom of Menopause, Creating Physical and Emotional Health During the Change* online or at an independent bookstore.

The Buzz on Bee Pollen

Bee Pollen Benefit-Rich in protein, lipids, minerals, phenolic compounds and vitamins, Bee Pollen has been recognized as an antifungal, antibacterial and antiviral agent that has a number of positive health effects. It is richer in protein than any other animal source. In a study done in 2005 by the Tokyo University of Agriculture, researchers found that bee pollen has a significant antioxidant activity. Another study done in Japan, in 2008, found that bee pollen may also be a natural allergy fighter. Leo Conway, MD in Denver, treated his patients with a bee pollen supplement. Those who took this supplement for three years remained allergy free throughout this time. Bee pollen is helpful in preventing some of the menopausal symptoms in women. The flavonoids that can be found in pollen also help prevent the breast cancer. It is one of the best supplements for stress and it proved to be particularly useful for people who suffer from a lack of energy. This makes bee pollen an especially great medicine for older adults. The consumption of bee pollen also helps reverse the signs of aging skin. It protects the skin from dehydration and helps increase the blood supply to the skin cells. Being rich in nucleic acids RNA and DNA, it serves as a rejuvenator for the skin. A Russian scientist, Naum Petrovich Ioyrish, author of the book *Bees and people*, believes that people who take bee pollen live longer. And doctor Lars Erik Essen from Sweden believes that the bee pollen has a number of important biological effects on the body that stops cells from premature aging.

- **Panax Ginseng** – A plant that has been used in traditional Chinese medicine for thousands of years, Panax ginseng reduces fatigue and endurance and increases energy. It balances hormones, improves appetite, and can alleviate symptoms of depression and anxiety. Some evidence also shows that continual usage of Panax ginseng can boost mental performance in people with Alzheimer's disease. In combination with gingko leaf extract, it can improve memory. According to some data by the University of Maryland Medical Center, Panax ginseng can help improve the overall immune system and stress resistance. The extract should be used for two to three weeks, followed by a two-week pause. The active complex of Panax ginseng can help restore the cellular function, therefore making it useful in anti-aging treatments too. This is especially true with Asian ginseng which is rich in antioxidants and insulin-like substances.

- **Royal Jelly** – Boasting a number of positive effects on health including increased circulation, prevention of premature aging, lowering blood pressure, and preventing certain types of cancer, Royal Jelly is rich in minerals such as calcium, iron, and potassium, but also vitamin B, nucleic acids, and seventeen amino acids. Some of the proteins that can be found in royal jelly have a direct effect on the blood pressure. Adding royal jelly to the diet also helps eliminate the bad cholesterol levels, therefore preventing a number of cardiovascular diseases such as heart attacks and strokes. The antioxidants and minerals that are found in royal jelly, can help fight off the free radicals, which cause the premature aging. These antioxidants are helpful in eliminating wrinkles by helping the skin produce more collagen, a study by the Department of East-West Medical Science of Kyung Hee University. One of the main proteins that can be found in royal jelly - MRJP1 is responsible for the production of collagen. Royal Jelly can slow or prevent macular degeneration and even hair loss. A study published in Advanced Biomedical Research showed that the royal jelly played a beneficial part in neural functions, and for that reason plays an important role in preventing and treating neurodegenerative disease such as the Alzheimer's. Royal Jelly can also help minimize the bad effects of menopause and act as a mood booster. Some studies have also shown that royal jelly can help with the issues associated with vaginal atrophy. Women who took royal jelly cream showed more improvement than those who were prescribed a lubricant or the vaginal estrogen cream. In combination with Gingko Biloba and Panax ginseng, royal jelly has been found to improve memory functions in older adults.

- **Spirulina** – A blue green algae that grows in freshwater. Ayurveda describes spirulina as capturing the energy of the sun. Spirulina boosts immunity, is good for heart health and the eyes. Spirulina slows aging and helps to boost energy. Spirulina also helps the body eliminate toxins. Nasa conducted studies on spirulina as a food for the future that could feed people in outer space.

Detox may also be needed if one is exposed to chemical hormone disruptors. If you suspect this is the case you may want to consult an LAc, a naturopath, and osteopath or a medical doctor specializing in detox. Avoid all plastics, microwaving in plastics (reference a few things from The Telomere Effect.)

Rasayanas

Rasayanas are traditional Indian herbal and food-based formulas, usually made into the form of a sweet paste. These formulas are designed to rejuvenate and slow the aging process at the deepest level. These nectarous superfoods are often prescribed in traditional Ayurvedic medicine. In fact, on my first trip to India, I went to a school of Ayurveda and was given a rasayana. I had no idea at the time what it was or how to take it. I took spoonfuls of the paste wondering what the strange brown paste was doing to me. Specific and synergistic herbs and foods are used for rasayana, creating herbal jams are help rebuild and enhance the quality of our tissues. These are the original longevity foods. There are seven tissues or *dhatus* (Sanskrit word for when we rejuvenate and rebuild our tissues), according to Ayurveda, this leads to stronger immunity and a longer life. Rasayana help to restore functions of the body that have become deficient, excessive or damaged. Rasayanas are also recommended before and after cleanses or detox regimens. In Ayurveda, a cleanse prepares a person to open up to receive good nutrition and rejuvenating therapies. Rasayanas restore the body and provide materials for rejuvenation.

- **Chyawanprash** – This an herbal paste made with honey and ghee that contains, a variety of herbs and berries, including, amla berry, ashwaghanda, wild asparagus, cardamom, tulsi, cinnamon, sesame oil, tulsi, ginger, and bacopa. Royal Physicians formulated this paste during Vedic times. High in vitamin C, Chyawanprash can be taken alone, with tea or spread on bread, crackers or fruit. Or take 1 tsp per day to build immunity, balance hormones and boost your energy.
- **Shilajit**-A trace mineral blend, combined with fulvic acid. This paste is prepared and taken as a traditional rasayana for detoxification. Take Shilajit in very small amounts mixed with tea, juice or water
- **Triphala** – A combination of three high antioxidant berries, triphala helps one to detox gently and naturally on a daily basis. You can take triphala as a powder, mixed with water to eliminate toxins from the body and to promote regular elimination.
- **Amrit Kalash** – In the 1980s, Maharishi Mahesh Yogi decided to create a rasayana to combat the stress of modern life. He gathered eminent Ayurvedic scholars and physicians to help create the formula which was named Amrit Kalash, giving it a nod to the legend of the Samudra Manthan in which the oceans are churned with herbs and gems to create a nectar of immortality. A few of the ingredients in Amrit Kalash

are Amla or Indian Gooseberry, Indian Gallnut, turmeric, long pepper, Gotu Kola, and Shankhpushpi More information at www.mapi.com

- **Hanah One** – Based on Chyawanprash, Hanah One is a modern rasayana that combines a traditional Ayurveda formula made in tasty base of ghee and honey along with a long list of medicinal herbs and superfoods. The paste tastes good and can be taken alone or spread on bread, fruit or added to a smoothie or tea. www.hanahlife.com

- **Shankhpushpi** – A tonic for the brain, memory and memory. Shankhpushpi can support sound sleep as one ages. Shankhpushpi supports the nervous system and benefits all types of people as they age.

- **Ashwagandha** – See above for hormone balancing, Ashwagandha is also considered a rasayana.

- **Shatavari** – *Asparagus racemosus* or Shatavari has been used as a reproductive tonic for males and females, a demulcent for the digestive system and as an adaptogen. It has been used for centuries in Ayurveda as a reproductive tonic for women. Compounds in Shatavari relieve symptoms of menopause, such as hot flashes, vaginal atrophy, irritability and irregular memory. As a demulcent for the digestive system, Shatavari soothes the mucous membranes which help normalize the balance of acidity in our bodies and promote a healthy inflammatory response in the intestines. Another of the many medicinal properties of Shatavari is also its calming effect on the nervous system. It calms and nourishes the nerves, brain and helps support the brain and body when dealing with insomnia, pain or spasms

Other individual herbs that are considered Rasayanas are *shilajit* (could be thought of as a single herbal substance).

- **Pippali Evening Primrose Oil** – Evening Primrose oil comes from the evening primrose plant and it is one of the best oils for slowing aging. This powerful oil has been used around the world for thousands of years to heal. Native Americans used it to heal wounds and digestive issues. Evening Primrose played a part in Greek mythology while Greeks thought it helped to chase away the effects of over indulgence. In Ayurveda, Evening Primrose is known by its Sanskrit name, Artavashamana. It's considered a rasayana, a substance that improves immunity and life essence and slows the aging process. A modern study showed that skin moisture, firmness and elasticity improved after subjects consumed evening primrose oil after only 12 weeks. It's strong antioxidant properties prevent wrinkles and it also has a natural hormone balancing effect. osteoporosis, rheumatoid arthritis, high cholesterol, heart disease and Alzheimer's disease among others. Evening primrose oil is rich in vitamins such as A, C, E and K. Evening primrose has been known to stimulate hair growth when taken internally or even applied topically directly to the scalp and hair. Some studies have shown a positive effect of evening primrose oil on rheumatoid arthritis. The participants of the study reported decreased joint point after applying the evening primrose oil. However, if you plan to try it out, it might take up to three months for benefits to appear.

- **Borage Oil** – It's high in Gamma Linolenic Acid, twice as much as evening primrose oil. GLA can't be made by the body, has many benefits and difficult to find from food. Borage oil is packed with macronutrients such as fiber, fats, and protein, but also vitamin A and C.

  For this reason, borage oil is a medicinal substance you can take, inside and out. GLA itself has heart health benefits, specifically it protects against atherosclerosis, heart attacks and stroke. Borage oil has been used in traditional medicine for hundreds of years and is best known for its anti-inflammatory effects. I that our bodies cannot produce on its own. Borage Oil has positive effects on bone loss and osteoporosis, skin disorders, rheumatoid arthritis pain, diabetes, inflammation etc. GLA from borage oil has been shown to be effective with arthritis disorders. A group of twenty-seven patients were given either borage oil or the control cotton seed oil for 6 months. Borage seed oil was highly effective, reducing a tender joint score by almost 50 percent and reducing the number of tender joints, as well as inflamed joints. Traditionally borage oil is often recommended along with the primrose oil supplements for their synergistic effect on reducing inflammation. It's safe to use, although there are some side effects that should be taken into consideration. Diarrhea and bloating can occur. People who're taking aspirin or blood thinning medications should avoid borage oil because it can act like a blood thinner. Sick of pills, try drizzling borage oil on salads and soups. Don't use borage oil to cook or heat it to a high temperature or it will destroy its medicinal properties.

- **Fennel** – contains an impressive array of phytochemical compounds. Use it whole or ground to flavor dishes. It stimulates digestive fire and helps alleviate gas and bloating. As a carminative herb it assists with peristalsis. Fennel balances female hormones and reduces inflammation.

VITAMINS AND NUTRIENTS

In general there are many, many vitamins and nutrients that you can buy to Super Age. Right here are just a few. I recommend that you take food-based vitamins, which means the dried, powdered and either encapsulated or formed into tablets of whole-food substances. Some brands that make whole-food vitamins are Mega Food, Garden of Life. There are also many powdered whole-food supplements that you can find and add to water or other liquids to make a nutrient-dense smoothie or shake.

- **Magnesium** – Known as an anti-stress mineral, magnesium helps to balance blood sugar, optimizes circulation, blood pressure and relaxes muscles, reduces pain and activates the parasympathetic nervous system to calm the body. Mark Hyman. According to a study in the

Journal of Intensive Care Medicine, one is twice as likely to die with a deficiency in the mineral magnesium. It can improve sleep, making it an uber critical mineral for Super Aging.

Magnesium can be found in sea vegetables, green leafy vegetables, parsley, buckwheat, avocado, spirulina, sesame seeds, Brazil nuts, beans or whole grains. Magnesium can also be absorbed transdermally by taking an epsom salt bath or by using a transdermal patch. Magnesium absorption through the intestines can be affected by stress, alcohol, sodas, antibiotics and other drugs. People with kidney or heart disease should only take magnesium supplements under a doctor's supervision. Magnesium can be taken as a whole-food supplement or in the form of magnesium citrate, or magnesium glycinate. The RDA is 300 mg per day, but Dr. Mark Hyman believes beneficial dosages to be around 400–1000 per day. The amount of magnesium in our food has declined 25–80 percent from the 1950s.

Take magnesium transdermally, gel or oil Ancient Magnesium makes a spray oil for the skin or has excellent quality bath salts.

- **Vitamin E and Tocotrienols** – Vitamin E has numerous benefits—from preventing heart diseases, balancing cholesterol, repairing damaged skin, balancing hormones and more.

A study in 2013 confirmed that vitamin E is the main contributor in upkeeping the estrogen level and offering relief from menopausal symptoms, hot flashes, palpitation, insomnia, dyspareunia, dizziness, and vaginal dryness. In their clinical trial, they divided fifty-two postmenopausal women into two groups. One group was using 100 IU of vitamin E and the second group was using estrogen cream over the course of twelve weeks.

Their finding found that even though estrogen cream was more effective, vitamin E improves the laboratory criteria for vaginal atrophy and treatment success. So, vitamin E is a great solution for women who are unable to use hormone therapy or cope with the associated side effects. Taking a combination of 400 IU of alpha-tocopherol with 400mg vitamin tocotrienols every day is an important part of controlling hot flashes. A study in Iran that gathered a group of women in menopause found that taking a certain dosage of vitamin E every day for four weeks reduced the average frequency of hot flashes from five a day to three, and made them less severe when they occured.

A study has shown that the specific A study has shown that the specific isomers of vitamin E successfully fight the cholesterol oxidation and prevents further damage to the body done by the free radicals. These isomers also help in slowing down the aging process as they fight off the free radicals, making vitamin E a strong antioxidant. Vitamin E is great for treating sunburns and in combination with vitamin C, it helps minimize the risk of exposure to the UV lights. Not only is it great for skin, but vitamin E has also found its use in hair products thanks to its moisturizing effects. In combination with vitamin C and zinc, vitamin E has shown to improve vision and decrease the macular degeneration that's related to aging. This same combination can also decrease risk of dementia in older people.

- **Tocotrienols:** Not many people are aware that vitamin E consists of eight different compounds. Half of these are called tocotrienols. Scientists have recently discovered that tocotrienols provide therapeutic and preventative options for aging. They reduce the risk of cancer and some of the most dangerous chronic diseases.

  Tocotrienols have presented an ability to inhibit the growth of new blood vessels to fast-growing tumors. They are also capable of sensitizing cancer cells to the effects of chemotherapy, combating cancer stem cells (which are resistant to chemo and contribute to cancer recurrences). In addition, tocotrienols are very effective when fighting cardiovascular diseases. They lower plasma cholesterol levels by blocking *HMG-CoA* reductase. This enzyme is a rate-limiting step in producing cholesterol, so blocking is means of lowering cholesterol levels.

Women who suffered hot flashes as consequences of cancer treatment also experienced some relief, although not as much.

PREVENTION IS THE BEST MEDICINE

Age-Related Macular Degeneration

Western medicine defines macular degeneration as incurable, yet there are many ways to prevent or slow age-related macular degeneration. As the main cause of irreversible vision loss among older adults, causing them slowly over time to lose their central vision. In time, a person with AMD will experience difficulties or find it impossible to drive, read, or recognize familiar faces.

Prevention of AMD – You Should Be Diligent About Taking All Steps

- Stop smoking
- Eat Omega three oils fish or taking fish oil supplement
- Exercising regularly and maintaining a healthy weight
- Increase fresh whole foods in diet, especially foods such as fresh greens and berries
- Limit your intake of high-glycemic index foods
- Wearing sunglasses to block UV and blue light that are known for causing eye damage

In addition, Ayurveda recommends the following herbs to help slow or prevent AMD. Take triphala tea or tablets, 500–1000 mg daily. Drink tulsi tea 1–3 cups daily or as often as possible.

Add 1–3 tsps. spirulina to a smoothie or juice, drink daily or take 1–3 tablets or capsules daily.

—PRACTICE PLAN—

Make Natural Medicines a Part of Your Super Aging Plan

Check with your Functional Medicine doctor, Herbalist, Naturopath, or LAc (Licensed Acupuncturist) to determine which supplements would support your health and lifestyle.

Have a Daily Plan

What do you drink/take in the morning? Make a habit of daily hydration. Drink warm water with lemon or herbal tea, every day without fail.

Midday

If you take supplements, they are best digested between 10–2, take them during this window of time for your body to assimilate and digest.

Evening

Take only supplements or teas that will relax you. And don't drink after a certain hour depending on what's best for you. You will want to avoid having to go to the bathroom after a certain hour because you won't want interrupted sleep from having to get up and urinate.

Having a routine of supportive teas, juices and some vitamins, medications. You will have your own program and as always ease into it. Sometimes it is good to take a break from certain medicines and supplements while others need to be taken every day for some people.

If you have never meditated before, use the habit trigger reward system to create a meditation habit. Example: Get out of bed. Sit in chair, meditate, reward, drink coffee. Or:

Trigger —> Drink tea (Habit) = Meditate (Reward) + read the paper, look at social media for five minutes, eat a yummy breakfast

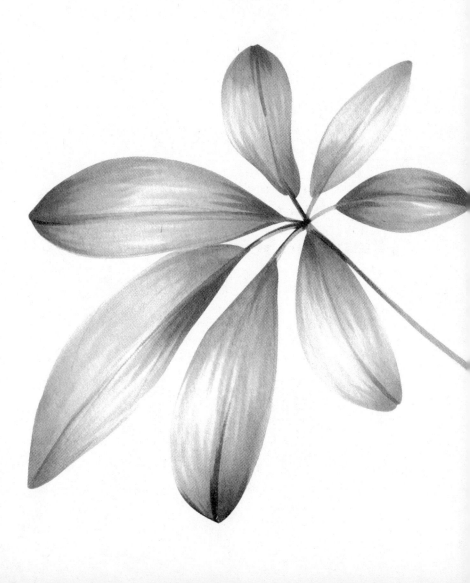

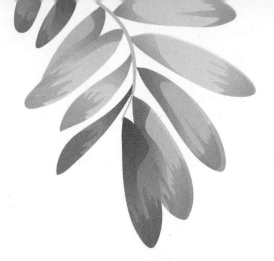

CHAPTER 13

Get Rid of the Weeds and Plant the Seeds for the Best Years of Your Life

> *"The heart is like a garden: it can grow compassion or fear, resentment or love."*
>
> —Jack Kornfield

PLANTING A GARDEN

You have a life you've already lived. You've developed preferences, inclinations, health histories, ways of being in relationship, a career or careers, habits, families, memories, and more. You have suffered, you've felt intense joys and sorrows. You have fallen in love and had your heart broken. As you age you have choices, yet not everyone sees the choices available in each moment, in each day, in each month and each year. You can limit your capacity to live the life you truly would like to live by giving up. You will have regrets and wasted years. You can wallow in loses and misunderstandings. Taking control of your life may sometimes feel daunting or impossible. When you are faced with setbacks such as cancer, loss of a spouse, illness or divorce, you may feel like giving up. Some days it may be good to just curl up in a ball. To be mindful is to feel the feelings, yet to have compassion for yourself and others. From that place a tiny seed grows. At first that seed seems small, over time it grows. Those little seeds are your daily habits. Plant these seeds for when times are tough, the weather or conditions are rough, you will lean into the habits that strengthen your body and your soul.

Motivation. At the core of your ability and inclination to age well is your reason for living, your motivation or your purpose. Use whatever word works for your life and your personality. If you are unclear about why you are here, go back to Chapter 2 and spend time daily, writing, meditating and pondering what brings you joy. What makes your soul sing? What deeply motivates you to show up for the hard stuff? Is it your grandchildren? Is it nature? Is it your business? Is it helping others? Refer back to Chapter 1 for more ways to tap into your purpose or reason for living.

Next you are going to put down a simple plan on paper. I encourage you to make this plan as visual as possible. If you can draw, wonderful. If not, grab some magazines or print some photos. The soul speaks through images. The more you create symbols for your Super Aging plan, the more powerful your plan will be. Remember you can plan to be as big and beautiful as you could ever imagine as you age. How will you do this? How can you change our life with just one brushstroke or one pill? One action only will not work, nor will one pill. When instead, you imagine your life as a garden, you will be ready to understand the steps it will take. A garden is the perfect metaphor, it takes time to grow. A garden may have been neglected, but it can always be replanted. Seeds planted today will bear fruit later. There are tasks that need to be done every day to create a beautiful garden.

CHANGING HABITS

Many people find changing habits difficult. You may have ways of thinking that you've held for so long. In the garden metaphor, you can plan what to grow and plant. It doesn't have to happen all at once. And once something begins to grow, it has its own momentum. You will feel a sense of proficiency and will more likely feel encouraged to make better choices going forward. Through the metaphor of a garden you can create a beautiful place for aging. You will realize that your life is more like a work of art, than something that just happens. You will initiate a new way of being and you will take control of your lives. It is powerful to take life into your own hands to live at any age, but especially as older adults.

Limiting Beliefs, these are the weeds. Many weeds actually are very nourishing. Weeds like dandelions and other "invasives" are edible and can help you heal. Right now, you are going to either make those weeds useful and nourishing or get rid of them. Weeds symbolize habits and practices in your life that need some alchemy. Either your outlook needs to change, or your habits need to change. Maybe some things will stay and will grow. Nourishing weeds that feel comfortable and that help you grow. Some you may want to give to others, either truly or metaphorically. Maybe you want to get rid of a lot of clutter. As you age you may find you acquire lots of stuff. As you age you may have outdated ways of behaving or habits that do not serve you. You may want to weed out junk food, late nates or gossiping friends to make room to plant a new career or take up a hobby, like playing the saxophone.

You may read *Super Ager* and think, wow it is cool to see all of these Super Agers and what they are doing. I feel inspired! And then you return to your life. But it takes more than inspiration to age well, you must take action to Super Age. You are in it for the long haul. Your goal is to take that fire of your purpose or reason for living and turn it into a representation of how you want to age. One step at a time, changing starts with daily habits, weekly habits and seasonal habits. When you plant a garden, you must water the garden daily. You must do weekly and monthly tasks. You will also have seasonal tasks. You are going to plant your life garden. When you have a plan, you can change your life and your lifestyle. Your life plan exists in harmony with you and nature. The resilience needed to Super Age is the resilience of a garden. Remember that our health as you age is determined largely by lifestyle, not (70–80 percent) not genetics. You have the ability to age well. You can wait for researchers to create an anti-aging pill, or mutant worm makeover. Cynthia Kenyon and her lab at UCSF were able to increase the lifespan of a little worm, *c. elegans*, by tenfold. Someday, maybe sooner or later, scientists may unlock some of the biological mechanisms that cause aging. Yet time marches on and even if aging becomes reversible, who knows. This book and your plan is really about living your life in harmony means living every day. When you live in balance with nature and who you are as an individual, you will live to the fullest. Life holds no guarantees. I do know that when you live in balance and harmony, you will feel more satisfied and hopeful. You will give to others, you will give to the world. Your life will be a contribution and you will not regret your choices. To live well is to keep your body in great shape. It does not mean you are perfect. It means you may have suffered health issues and you now take care of yourself to the best of your ability, mind, body and spirit. If you have had an accident or injury, you can practice meditation, you can pray if it feels right.

PRUNING BAD HABITS

Cutting away the old can be painful. When you experience the pain of change at any age, think of it as weakness leaving the body. The best way to start changing is to begin with low-hanging branches. Take out the habits that are easiest to fix. Perhaps you can start by taking one less bite of junk food. That sounds incredibly silly, but it is a start. If you eat a candy bar every day, try throwing away the last bite. Do this for a week. If you aren't successful, keep doing this exercise until you are then trying to leave two bites. Keep doing this until you stop eating candy bars. By starting small, you eliminate a bad habit one bite at a time.

To add in good habits, think of it as planting seeds, you will plant a seed for adding more vegetables into your diet. Start small, add three extra servings a week or eat one more vegetable a day. Make it so easy you can't say no. You could try just a few eating carrot sticks every day. Then add an extra serving of greens once a week. You will often find that this slow and gradual approach helps you gain slow, but powerful momentum. Soon you will be eating far more vegetables than you ever imagined.

As for right now, you will need to take care of yourself. Dr. Dale Bredesen works with his patients on a strict protocol that loosely similar to many of the lifestyle recommendations of Super Ager. His patients are facing an Alzheimer's diagnosis, so they need to work quickly to reverse the damage already taking hold in their brains. His patients need to quickly adopt the ReCode protocol. While there may or may not be urgency in how you adopt and change your own lifestyle to create and optimize your own aging, I like the idea of thinking of yourself as an elite athlete. While many of the Super Agers stories contained in this book are about people who may not have expected to live such a long and incredible lives, many Super Agers do tend to have disciplined and conscientious habits. The good news is that you decide what will work best for you right now. What would be the easiest thing to change in your life? What habit or lifestyle shift would you be able to make right now? Flip through the pages, look at the daily and weekly habits. And then decide. The founder of Yoga Health Coaching, Cate Stillman taught me to teach people to look for the low-hanging fruit. When you change something easily, you start to gain momentum and feel hopeful about making other positive changes in our lives.

Start by committing to one small change. For example, your change could be meditating for one minute every day. You want the change to be so small you can't say no to at least trying it. Maybe for you it could start with walking for ten minutes every day. If that is too long, what about five minutes or even two minutes, you just want to jumpstart that *habit*. To change your diet, start by spending fifteen minutes, one day a week, meal planning. Planning your meals can have an incredible cascading effect on your food consumption, so a fifteen-minute planning session could reap incredible rewards. Maybe your commitment could be to start to climbing stairs when you see them. Whenever you have the opportunity to take the elevator or stairs, commit to stairs and allow extra them. Once you accomplish this first habit change and you have made it a habit for twenty-one to thirty days. Go to the next section of your garden and begin a new habit. It works really well to do this with a group or at least one buddy. It can be easy to give up or over think things, talking over your plans and committing to them with a friend, mentor or group can make all the difference.

SETTING GOALS

The remarkable thing about people who age well and live 100 years. They are always setting goals. Goals help our minds to grow and look ahead. Goals help our physiology and help us tap into the continuity of time. Bhagvan Kani, 115 years old would like to preside over his great, great granddaughters wedding. Even though he is 115, he sets goals for his future. Doreetha Daniels wanted to graduate from community college, even though she suffered several strokes while she was enrolled in school in Santa Clarita, CA. She stuck to her goal of graduating before she turned 100 years of age and graduated at age 99. Your goals inspired others. The lives you will touch with your goals and dreams will inspire your students, your coworkers, your family, and your community. The goals you set from fifty onward help others to dream, to imagine, to believe in a world that can be different.

What is the next seed you want to plant? Do you want to exercise? Do you want to add more plants to your diet? Do you want more fun or play? more friendships. Take it slow. Pick one thing to change at a time. A tiny habit is a nudge. Move slowly, change becomes doable, when you break things in to tiny bite size habits. If you feel overwhelmed flip a coin or write your choices down and just pick only one thing. Really the decision is more important than perfection, so when all else fails flip a coin or just pick something, it is always the right choice.

Each day we plant seeds each day we water seeds, we fertilize, we tear out old plants, and we must think of her life in this way it's not about one pill one pill would be like just doing one thing in the garden sometimes our lives are complicated, and we may need help from a master gardener (medical professional). Self-care and healthy lifestyle habits are an art based on science and informed by tradition. Each one of us lives only in the moment, yet in each moment exists the choice to grow or cut back. Like a garden, we can choose to slowly grow the life-affirming habits and personal qualities that will help us to live healthy and satisfying lives. No guarantees exist in life, but we do have this choice, each day, each hour an opportunity to grow and change to create a legacy.

Health coach at Yoga Health Coach in fact we may need many helpers many gardeners along the way yet we can also do a lot on her own shouldn't be up just to the master gardeners some people may prefer this it's best to learn what we can do and how we can upkeep the garden on her own how can we take care of what we planted what do we need to do what I'm suggesting is to make a plan this may mean contacting a nutritionist, an acupuncturist, a medical doctor

Get ready to make a visual representation of your plan to Super Age.

Grab a Pen and Paper

Create a Garden Map. Your garden can have any shape you like, just make sure you keep the following idea in mind. The feng shui of your mind is loosely based on the idea that, as you plant things, each new addition shifts the entire outline And if your garden shifts when you plant one thing, other things will pop up; some may need to be weeded out and some may need to be planted again—until it looks unrecognizable from how you started. Keep this in mind.

Now it's time to put together a plan. A landscape map that will help you right now to become a Super Ager. The fun part is that you have been working towards this plan your entire life. This landscape plan is designed for you to have more fun, more joy, enjoy what you love, to feel and look great.

Start with your overall goals or "big picture" garden plans. Some things that will affect the entire garden are mindset, meditation, and purpose. You can mark areas to develop these tools in your garden for the actual actions of meditating, journaling, or other activities. But think of your mindset as the soil. You are going to add some mulch. Perhaps this means composting some old beliefs:

- Write the old beliefs down
- Get rid of worry
- Let go of controlling behavior (stop telling your kids what to do)
- Reduce complaining
- Reframe anger
- Let go of lost years, being married to the wrong person, being in the wrong career

When creating your plan, do what makes sense, what comes naturally, what you enjoy. Check in with your gut, your intuition. Your plan is unique and it's all about you.

TOP PRIORITIES

Find Your Purpose

Motivation. Your purpose or ikigai. If these feel weak, it's time to rekindle the fire of your ambition. Your purpose or reason for living can be very simple and fluid. Let go of ego, this fire comes from a burning desire. What makes you sing with joy? Never what gets others attention or is a distraction to prop you up when you have low self-esteem. If you find you are feeling less than optimal about yourself, add the following to your garden: practices that boost neurogenesis, exercise (which should always be number one), and meditation, which has been shown to help with purpose. Boosting your self-worth will in turn help you uncover that ikigai that has been temporarily dormant or long dormant. When your health becomes stronger and your creative juices are flowing, your purpose may be shining through.

Create Your Vision

American Olympian Nastia Liukin won five gold medals and she believes in "vision boards." "Something I've always done while training and continue to do now is that every New Year's Eve, I sit down and make a new vision board for the year," she says. "I jot down my goals, things I want to accomplish, places I want to visit, etc. I also make it a fun project by adding motivational quotes, stickers, you name it."

Make sure creating your vision board is fun. When we do things with emotion, we create memories. We are creating neural pathways into the future. Some people like to make vision boards alone, some prefer to make them with a friend, spouse or group of likeminded people. Making vision boards can be fun and productive especially when you tie the creation of your vision with a birthday, new year's or a vacation or retreat. It makes a fun and entertaining group activity for a party or group event.

A vision board offers an easy visual target to help your lifestyle changes to stay on track. Athletes have taken to this strategy because research backs up the efficacy of visualization. A 2004 study, one group of participants went to the gym for regular training sessions, another group was asked to simply visualize the training sessions and a control group was asked to do nothing. The visualizing group made 50 percent of the muscle gains of the gym going group. Scientists concluded that combining workouts with visualizations make training much easier. Why not try visualization as you age?

One little rosebush in one corner we need to care for the overall garden water weed prune out so many things are going to take care of that garden and that's what you're going to need to do in order to choose that you need to choose positivity and compassion for yourself your face adversity as your age so it's imperative that you latch onto this growth mindset yes

The most important takeaway from this book could be that you can develop your own healthy relationship to the aging process. Research and advice will continue to accumulate exponentially on what will make for a healthy aging process. The most important question remains, what works best for you? And what will work best for you right now? What do you feel will help you and your family as you age? Journaling will also be addressed as in addition to collaging and drawing journaling can be an indispensable way to get in touch with what feels right for you in your life and aging process. Grab your journal and begin to brain storm, what plants do you want to get rid of? What weeds that are no longer helping you would you like to pull? What weeds are actually powerful and helpful that might be better to keep? Look at the list of areas to grow. Imagine each area is a place in your garden. What would you plant or prune back? What seeds or new habits do you want to plan. Give your garden plan a time line.

-PLAN YOUR VISION-

Prepare Your Super Ager Vision Board

You will need paper. This can be an unlined notebook, a blank sheet of 8½ by 11-inch printer paper, or a larger piece of paper from a craft store or local drugstore.

Decide if you will make a collage or draw. Get magazines for collaging or get colorful pencils or markers for drawing. Make it fun and use supplies that inspire you.

Make Your Super Ager Vision Board

1. Go through the areas you want to develop right now. Some examples are:
   - Meditations/Spirituality
   - Nourishment/Food
   - Community
   - Body/Exercise
   - Mindful Mindset
   - Healthy Brain
   - Purpose
   - Calm

2. Determine what you need to do in order to get there and feel free to add these to your board.

3. Post your vision board somewhere you can view it often.

4. Review and/or add to it every so often to jeep your vision fresh!

LIVE IN HARMONY WITH NATURE

Extend your life and change your habits to become a Super Ager. Place your hand on your heart, breathe in deeply. Give yourself a surge of compassion. Give yourself some more. You have lived a life. It isn't always easy so treat yourself kindly. Put out your best effort and let go of the results. Longevity is 75 percent lifestyle so make your lifestyle fun and healthy. Choose healthy habits so you can live the life to the fullest. Balanced living is key. Super Agers embrace life, living in the moment, with intrinsic purpose. Super Agers share their lives with close friends and family, surrounding themselves with likeminded individuals who support and nurture the life that they have chosen. Super Agers choose joy in the face of setbacks.

Live in harmony with nature in a way that honors your true nature, you are a Super Ager. It is your birthright to Super Age. In the end it is never about a number, but the legacy and love you leave behind, no matter your years. I hope you have found inspiration to live by the principles of Super Agers. The more we spread the values of Super Aging, we will leave the world a better place.

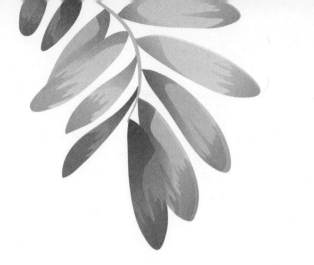

REFERENCES

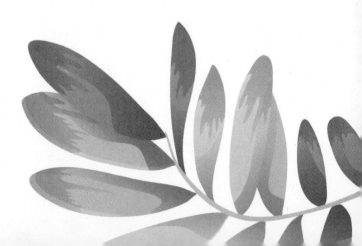

Apfel, Iris Barrel. *Iris Apfel: Accidental Icon*. New York, NY: Harper Design, 2018.

Blackburn, Elizabeth, and Elissa Epel. *The Telomere Effect: A Revolutionary Approach to Living Younger, Healthier, Longer*. New York: Grand Central Publishing, 2018.

Bredesen, Dale E. *The End of Alzheimer's: The First Program to Prevent and Reverse Cognitive Decline*. New York: Avery, 2017.

Chaudhary, Kulreet, and Eve Adamson. *The Prime: Prepare and Repair Your Body for Spontaneous Weight Loss*. New York: Harmony Books, 2016.

Collins, Elise Marie. *An A–Z Guide to Healing Foods: A Shopper's Reference*. Berkeley, CA: Conari Press, 2010.

Cortright, Brant. *The Neurogenesis Diet and Lifestyle: Upgrade Your Brain, Upgrade Your Life*. Mill Valley (CA): Psyche Media, 2015.

Garcia, Hector. *Ikigai: The Japanese Secret to a Long and Happy Life*. Penguin Books, 2017.

Garcia, Hector, and Francesc Miralles. *Ikigai: The Japanese Secret to a Long and Happy Life*. Penguin Books, 2017.

Helft, Miguel. "Meet Forward, An Ex-Googler's Plan To Reinvent Health Care With A Dose Of Apple, Netflix And AI." *Forbes*, January 17, 2017.

Keeling, Ida, and Anita Doreen Diggs. *Can't Nothing Bring Me Down: Chasing Myself in the Race against Time*. Grand Rapids, MI: Zondervan, 2018.

LaPallo, Bernardo. *Age Less, Live More*. Perfect Paperback, 2009.

Needham, Belinda L., Judith E. Carroll, Ana V. Diez Roux, Annette L. Fitzpatrick, Kari Moore, and Teresa E. Seeman. *Neighborhood Characteristics and Leukocyte Telomere Length: The Multi-Ethnic Study of Atherosclerosis.* Journal of Health and Place. July 2014.

Northrup, Christiane. *The Wisdom of Menopause: Creating Physical and Emotional Health and Healing During the Change.* New York: Bantam Books, 2001.

Porchon-Lynch, Tao, Janie Sykes Kennedy, and Teresa Kay-Aba Kennedy. *Dancing Light: The Spiritual Side of Being Through the Eyes of a Modern Yoga Master.* New York: Power Living Media, 2015.

Stevenson, Shawn. *Sleep Smarter: 21 Essential Strategies to Sleep Your Way to a Better Body, Better Health, and Bigger Success.* Emmaus, PA: Rodale, 2016.

Stillman, Cate. Body Thrive: *Uplevel Your Body and Your Life with 10 Habits from Ayurveda and Yoga.* Tetonia, ID: Yogahealer Press, 2015.

Super Centenarians, The Spice Mountains of Southwestern India. Directed by Murali Nair. 2014.

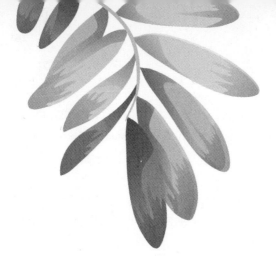

ABOUT THE AUTHOR

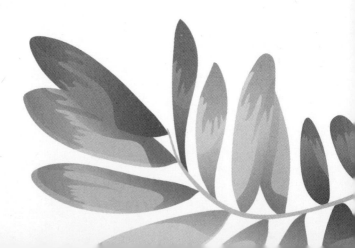

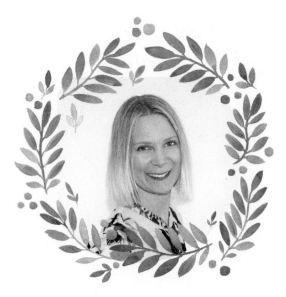

Elise Marie Collins is a visionary yoga teacher and health coach living in San Francisco. Elise's writing combines her love of ancient healing arts and scientific inquiry. She is currently instructing participants in a program on the effects of restorative yoga and stretching for metabolic syndrome. She's the author of *Super Ager*, *Chakra Tonics*, and Essential *Elixirs for Mind, Body and Spirit and An A-Z Guide to Healing Foods: A Shoppers Companion*. She has taught thousands to relax, eat well, move, breathe, and age well with yoga and motivational coaching.